Soft Tissue Reconstruction of the Hand: Loco-regional and Distant Flaps Selection and Approach

Obaid Almeshal • Salah Aldekhayel
Feras Alshomer
Editors

Soft Tissue Reconstruction of the Hand: Loco-regional and Distant Flaps Selection and Approach

Springer

Editors
Obaid Almeshal
Division of Plastic Surgery, Department of Surgery, King Abdulaziz Medical City
Ministry of National Guard - Health Affairs. King Abdullah International Medical Research Center
Riyadh, Saudi Arabia

Feras Alshomer
Division of Plastic Surgery, Department of Surgery, King Abdulaziz Medical City
Ministry of National Guard - Health Affairs. King Abdullah International Medical Research Center
Riyadh, Saudi Arabia

Salah Aldekhayel
Division of Plastic Surgery, Department of Surgery, King Abdulaziz Medical City
College of Medicine, King Saud bin Abdulaziz University for Health Sciences Ministry of National Guard - Health Affairs. King Abdullah International Medical Research Center
Riyadh, Saudi Arabia

ISBN 978-981-16-9947-4 ISBN 978-981-16-9945-0 (eBook)
https://doi.org/10.1007/978-981-16-9945-0

This Springer imprint is published by the registered company Springer Nature Singapore Pte Ltd.
The registered company address is: 152 Beach Road, #21-01/04 Gateway East, Singapore 189721, Singapore

This book is dedicated to the outstanding teamwork that made this work possible. All of your hard work has paid off.

Special thanks to my family, my wife, and my kids

Preface

It has been a sincere privilege to write and edit this book directed toward hand, plastic, and reconstructive surgeons. It addresses different levels of expertise ranging from medical students interested in the field to expert hand surgeons.

Most of the books and articles related to this field are either quite extensive and do not show the clinical scenario being managed or tunneled to the problem being discussed. This will lead to ambiguity and unclarity of the problem being managed, especially for young surgeons.

In this book, the reader will learn the different solutions related to hand soft tissue coverage options presented in an anatomical fashion and well-illustrated figures followed by a case scenario. The book was written in a bullet point fashion that discusses flap selection in easy-to-follow surgical steps, including postoperative instructions. The book will provide the reader with a solution related to hand soft tissue coverage that avoids the need for challenging microvascular skills.

Riyadh, Saudi Arabia | Obaid Almeshal, MBBS, SB-Plast

Acknowledgments

Special thanks are due to Dr. Abdullah Al-Thunayan, Dr. Abdullah Al-Namla and Professor Mohammad Al-Qattan, who provided unlimited support and had a tremendous impact as great mentors. Additionally, many thanks to Dr. Hanan Alhusainan who participated in the management and care of the patients.

Contents

Part III Finger-Related Flaps

Part IV Thumb-Related Flaps

Editors and Contributors

About the Editors

Obaid Almeshal, MBBS, SB-Plast Dr. Almeshal is a plastic and reconstructive surgeon with over 20 years' experience. As an editor of the book, Dr. Almeshal holds a subspecialty fellowship in brachial plexus and upper extremity reconstruction. He also focuses on hand surgery and reconstructive microsurgery in which he has authored multiple publications with remarkable contribution in this field.

Salah Aldekhayel, MBBS, FRCSC Dr. Aldekhayel is a senior plastic and reconstructive surgeon who co-edited this book. Dr. Aldekhayel has a keen interest in hand surgery and microvascular reconstruction in which he holds his subspecialty fellowship in. He has published numerous publications in the field of hand and reconstructive surgery with significant impact.

Feras Alshomer, MBBS, MSc, SB-Plast, JMC-PRS Dr. Alshomer is a board-certified plastic and reconstructive surgeon in which he co-edited this book. Dr. Alshomer has an extensive research and clinical experience with an interest in reconstructive microsurgery in which he has received his subspecialty training in. He has authored numerous book chapters and research papers with significant impact.

Contributors

Hassan abbas Ali Plastic Surgery Division, Department of Surgery, Ministry of National Guard - Health Affairs. King Abdullah International Medical Research Center, Riyadh, Saudi Arabia

Abdullaziz S. Alazzam, MBBS Plastic Surgery Division, Department of Surgery, Ministry of National Guard - Health Affairs. King Abdullah International Medical Research Center, Riyadh, Saudi Arabia

Salah Aldekhayel, MBBS, FRCSC Division of Plastic Surgery, Department of Surgery, King Abdulaziz Medical City, College of Medicine, King Saud bin Abdulaziz University for Health Sciences Ministry of National Guard - Health Affairs. King Abdullah International Medical Research Center, Riyadh, Saudi Arabia

Mohammed Alfawzan, MBBS, SB-Plast Plastic Surgery Division, Department of Surgery, Ministry of National Guard - Health Affairs. King Abdullah International Medical Research Center, Riyadh, Saudi Arabia

Turki Alhassan, MBBS, SB-Plast, JMC-PRS Plastic Surgery Division, Department of Surgery, Ministry of National Guard - Health Affairs. King Abdullah International Medical Research Center, Riyadh, Saudi Arabia

Bushra Alhazmi, MBBS Plastic Surgery Division, Department of Surgery, Ministry of National Guard - Health Affairs. King Abdullah International Medical Research Center, Riyadh, Saudi Arabia

Abdulaziz Alhujayri, MBBS, SB-Plast, JMC-PRS Plastic Surgery Division, Department of Surgery, Ministry of National Guard - Health Affairs. King Abdullah International Medical Research Center, Riyadh, Saudi Arabia

Hanan Alhusainan, MBBS, SB-Plast Plastic Surgery Division, Department of Surgery, Ministry of National Guard - Health Affairs. King Abdullah International Medical Research Center, Riyadh, Saudi Arabia

Obaid Almeshal, MBBS, SB-Plast Division of Plastic Surgery, Department of Surgery, King Abdulaziz Medical City, Ministry of National Guard - Health Affairs. King Abdullah International Medical Research Center, Riyadh, Saudi Arabia

Nawaf Alohaideb, MBBS, SB-Plast Plastic Surgery Division, Department of Surgery, Ministry of National Guard - Health Affairs. King Abdullah International Medical Research Center, Riyadh, Saudi Arabia

Malak Alsaif, MBBS Plastic Surgery Division, Department of Surgery, Ministry of National Guard - Health Affairs. King Abdullah International Medical Research Center, Riyadh, Saudi Arabia

Feras Alshomer, MBBS, MSc, SB-Plast, JMC-PRS Division of Plastic Surgery, Department of Surgery, King Abdulaziz Medical City, Ministry of National Guard - Health Affairs. King Abdullah International Medical Research Center, Riyadh, Saudi Arabia

Abdualziz S. Alshunaifi, MBBS Plastic Surgery Division, Department of Surgery, Ministry of National Guard - Health Affairs. King Abdullah International Medical Research Center, Riyadh, Saudi Arabia

Ahmed T. Al Turki, BScRC, MBBS, MSc Plastic Surgery Division, Department of Surgery, Ministry of National Guard - Health Affairs. King Abdullah International Medical Research Center, Riyadh, Saudi Arabia

Anas M. Alyamani, MBBS Plastic Surgery Division, Department of Surgery, Ministry of National Guard - Health Affairs. King Abdullah International Medical Research Center, Riyadh, Saudi Arabia

Ezekwe E. Amirize, MBBCh, FWACS, FICS, RCSEd Plastic Surgery Division, Department of Surgery, Ministry of National Guard - Health Affairs, King Abdullah International Medical Research Center, Riyadh, Saudi Arabia

Asmaa Z. Bin Mahmoud, MBBS Plastic Surgery Division, Department of Surgery, Ministry of National Guard - Health Affairs. King Abdullah International Medical Research Center, Riyadh, Saudi Arabia

Maher Elnahas, MBBS, MSc Plastic Surgery Division, Department of Surgery, Ministry of National Guard - Health Affairs, King Abdullah International Medical Research Center, Riyadh, Saudi Arabia

Ali I. Hadadi, MBBS Plastic Surgery Division, Department of Surgery, Ministry of National Guard - Health Affairs. King Abdullah International Medical Research Center, Riyadh, Saudi Arabia

Syed M. Ammar Yasir Jaffry, MBBS, MRCSEd, FCPS (Plast) Plastic Surgery Division, Department of Surgery, Ministry of National Guard - Health Affairs, Riyadh, Saudi Arabia

Muhammad Majid Ul Haq, FCPS plastic Plastic Surgery Division, Department of Surgery, Ministry of National Guard - Health Affairs, Riyadh, Saudi Arabia

Hazqeel Solangi, MBBS Plastic Surgery Division, Department of Surgery, Ministry of National Guard - Health Affairs, King Abdullah International Medical Research Center, Riyadh, Saudi Arabia

Part I

Random Flaps

Z-Plasty Flap and Its Variants

1

Bushra Alhazmi and Mohammed Alfawzan

Classification [1] Random flap, a triangular double transposition flap.

Vascular Supply [2] Subdermal plexus.

Innervation NA.

Indication [1, 3]
- To elongate tissue (i.e., a contracted linear scar)
- To break up a straight scar or to reorient a scar line for better alignment with relaxed skin tension lines (RSTL)
- To narrow the transverse axis of a scar.

Contraindications [2]
- Crush injury
- Local infection
- Extensive scarring of the area.

Advantages [1, 3, 4]
- It is a relatively simple procedure.
- There is no excision of normal tissue.
- It provides elongation along the axis of the central limb at the expense of shortening the perpendicular axis. The extent of tissue elongation is proportional to the angle of the flap (Table 1.1).

B. Alhazmi · M. Alfawzan (✉)
Plastic Surgery Division, Department of Surgery, Ministry of National Guard - Health Affairs, King Abdullah International Medical Research Center, Riyadh, Saudi Arabia

O. Almeshal et al. (eds.), *Soft Tissue Reconstruction of the Hand: Loco-regional and Distant Flaps Selection and Approach*,
https://doi.org/10.1007/978-981-16-9945-0_1

Table 1.1 Relation between Z-plasty lateral and central limb angle and percentage gained length

Angle degree	Percentage gained length
30°	25%
45°	50%
60°	75%
75°	100%
90°	120%

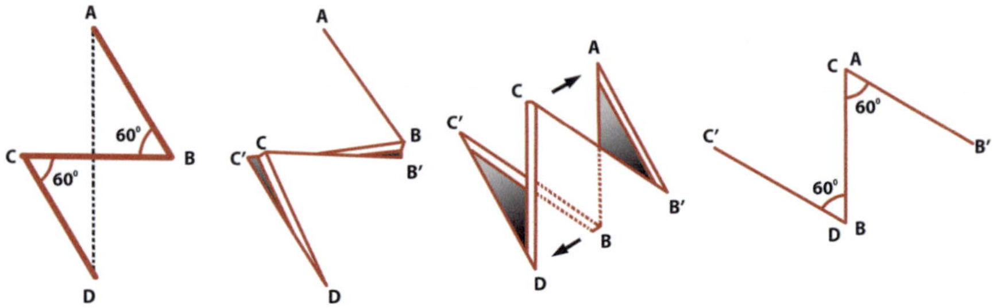

Fig. 1.1 The design and steps of Z-plasty are shown. From left to right, the Z-plasty was drawn with 60-degree angles with the central limb drawn over the scarred area. The two triangular flaps were raised with enough thickness and transposed. The final scar will be perpendicular to the original central limb of the Z-plasty

Disadvantages [1]

- It results in two additional scars.
- Wider flaps are more difficult to transpose.

Marking Technique [1, 3–5]

- In classic Z-plasty, the central limb is marked along the line of tension or the long axis of a scar.
- Two limbs are drawn at an equal angle to the central limb (i.e., 60 degrees) (Fig. 1.1).
- Several techniques have been described to facilitate the desired angle measurement [6].
- It is important to ensure that the length of the lateral limbs is equal to that of the central limb; otherwise, puckering at the corners and difficulty in closure will ensue.
- For each Z-plasty, two designs of the Z are possible. Usually, the one that results in better scar alignment with the RSTL is chosen.

Surgical Technique [1, 3–5]

- Following local, regional, or general anesthesia, prepping and draping of the surgical site are done in the usual sterile manner.
- An incision is made through the skin and subcutaneous tissue along the marked lines, using a no. 15 scalpel blade.
- Elevation of full-thickness skin flap is carried out with undermining at the level of subcutaneous fat, resulting in two triangular flaps of equal size.
- Some undermining of the adjacent subcutaneous tissue is done to facilitate mobilization of the flaps.

- Hemostasis is secured.
- The two triangular flaps are then raised and transposed around each other (Fig. 1.1).
- Tension-free skin closure is done in one layer using simple interrupted sutures.
- Topical antibiotics and firm pressure dressing are applied.

Postop Care [5]
- The wound is inspected 1–2 days postop.
- Suture removal, if needed, is done 7–14 days postop.

Complications [5]
- Hematoma
- Venous congestion
- Wound dehiscence
- Wound infection
- Partial flap necrosis
- Trapdoor effect.

Variants [3]
Many variations include but are not limited to the following:

- Compound Z-plasty (contiguous or interrupted). Refer to Fig. 1.2.
- Z-plasty with asymmetric angles

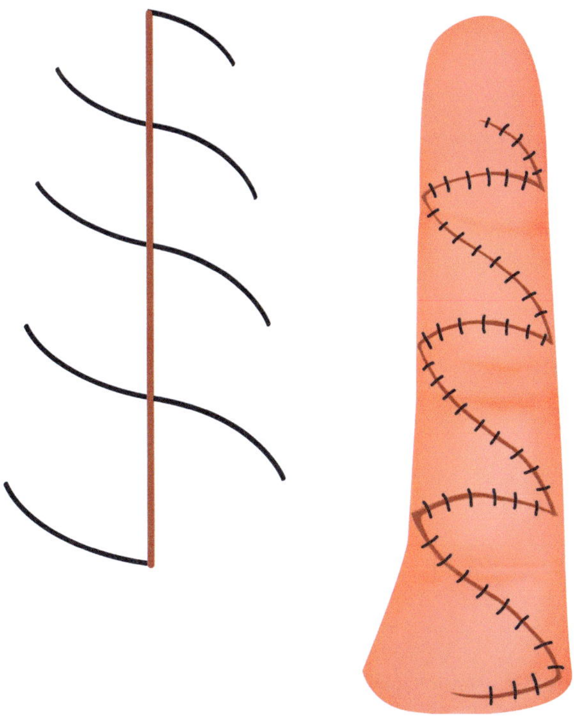

Fig. 1.2 Z-plasty can be drawn in a series of multiple continuous Z-plasties. This can give a wide exposure and is proved to be beneficial in certain conditions as in Dupuytren's contracture

- The three-flap Z-plasty [7]
- The double-opposing Z-plasty (butterfly flap)
- The four-flap Z-plasty: see next topic
- Star plasty
- The five-flap Z-plasty (jumping man flap) (refer to Fig. 1.3):
  - This modification consists of a central V-Y advancement flap and two lateral Z-plasties [8]. It is commonly used in the hand for interdigital web space contractures. It has also been described for digital flexion contracture [9]. The flap is marked as follows [8]:
    - The base limb is marked along the full length of the web.
    - The V flap limbs are drawn on the surface of more mobile tissue (palmar or dorsal depending on the individual case) with an angle of 60 degrees.
    - A straight limb is drawn starting at the apex of the V-Y flap extending to the opposite side of the base limb. This line represents the amount of advancement in the V-Y procedure. The length of advancement line is equal to the individual limbs of the V flap.
    - The Z-plasties are complete by drawing two equal lines at the proximal and distal ends of the base limb, respectively, at an angle of 80 degrees. Each Z-plasty will, therefore, have unequal angles of 80 degrees and 60 degrees.
    - The V-Y flap is advanced and the Z-plasty flaps on either side are transposed. The cumulative interdigitation of all flaps will result in a zigzag scar, as shown in Fig. 1.3.

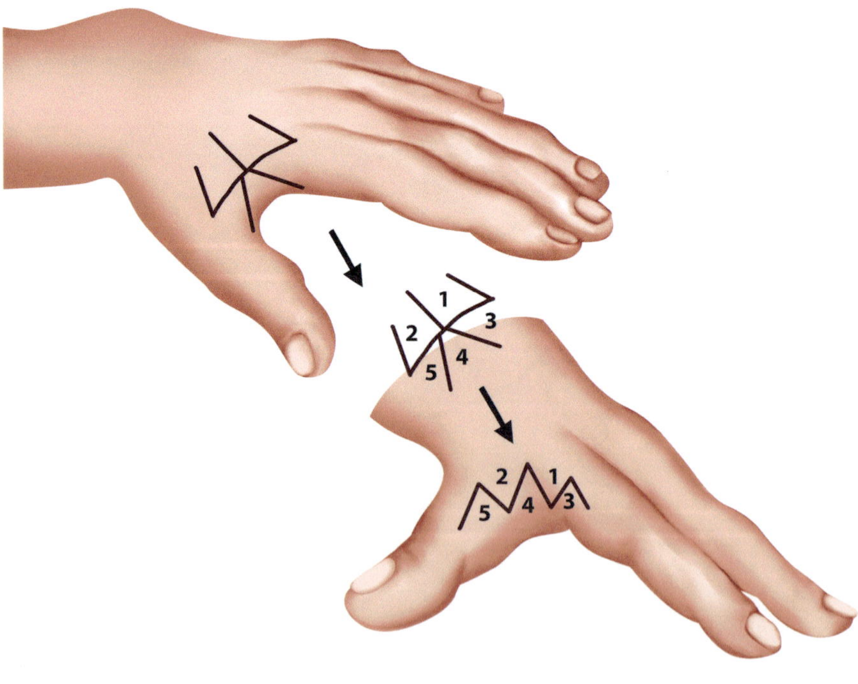

Fig. 1.3 The design of the jumping man flap is an excellent choice to deepen the contracted first web space of the hand. It is composed of 2 lateral Z-plasties joined in the middle with a V-Y flap. The two wide triangular flaps of the Z-plasties become more central next to the advanced V-Y flap

Case

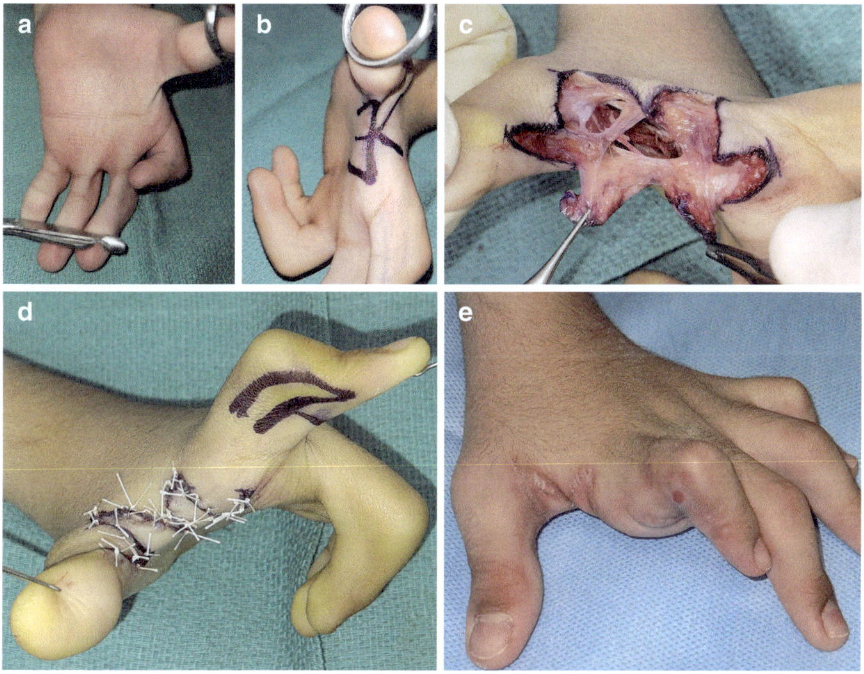

Case 1.1 Intraoperative photo of a patient who presented with first web space contracture in (**a**). The release of contracture was planned with the jumping man flap in which it was marked as seen in (**b**). After the skin incision, the flaps were raised, as seen in (**c**). The flaps were then transposed to their presumed location and the wounds were primarily closed, as shown in (**d**). After ensuring the proper release of the contracted thumb webspace, the follow-up assessment at 2 months is shown in (**e**) with maintained webspace

References

1. Shockley WW. Scar revision techniques: z-plasty, w-plasty, and geometric broken line closure. Facial Plast Surg Clin North Am. 2011 Aug;19(3):455–63.
2. Rehim S, Chung K. Local flaps of the hand. Hand Clin. 2014;30(2):137–51.
3. Hundeshagen G, Zapata-Sirvent R, Goverman J, Branski LK. Tissue rearrangements: the power of the Z-plasty. Clin Plast Surg. 2017 Oct;44(4):805–12.
4. McGregor IA. The Z-plasty in hand surgery. J Bone Joint Surg Br. 1967 Aug;49(3):448–57.
5. Salam GA, Amin JP. The basic Z-plasty. Am Fam Physician. 2003 Jun 1;67(11):2329–32.
6. Görgülü T, Olgun A. TG (tri-goniometry) technique: obtaining perfect angles in Z-plasty planning with a simple ruler. Burns. 2016 Mar;42(2):243–5.
7. Huang C, Ogawa R. Three-dimensional reconstruction of scar contracture-bearing axilla and digital webs using the Square Flap method. Plast Reconstr Surg Glob Open. 2014;2(5):e149.
8. Hirshowitz B, Karev A, Rousso M. Combined double Z-plasty and Y-V advancement for thumb web contracture. Hand. 1975 Oct;7(3):291–3.
9. Hashem AM. Use of the 5-flap Z plasty in digital flexion contractures. Ann Plast Surg. 2009 Nov;63(5):503–6.

Four-Flap Z-Plasty

2

Bushra Alhazmi and Mohammed Alfawzan

Classification [1] Random flap, a variation of Z-plasty.

Vascular Supply Subdermal plexus.

Innervation NA.

Indication [1–3]
- Lengthening of linear contracture
- Webspace deepening
- Classically used in contracture release and deepening of first webspace of the hand.

Contraindications [4]
- Crush injury
- Local infection
- Extensive scarring of the webspace
- Adduction contracture of the first metacarpal.

Advantages [1, 2]
- It is a simple procedure.
- It provides considerable length in areas where mobility is restricted due to severe contracture, such as webspaces, especially where a classic 60° Z-plasty is insufficient.

B. Alhazmi · M. Alfawzan (✉)
Plastic Surgery Division, Department of Surgery, Ministry of National Guard - Health Affairs, King Abdullah International Medical Research Center, Riyadh, Saudi Arabia

O. Almeshal et al. (eds.), *Soft Tissue Reconstruction of the Hand: Loco-regional and Distant Flaps Selection and Approach*,
https://doi.org/10.1007/978-981-16-9945-0_2

- Theoretically, a 100% and 150% increase in length of the central limb is gained with a 45° and 60° four-flap Z-plasty, respectively.
- It can result in up to 2 cm deepening of the first webspace (plus minimal muscle recession if required).

Marking Technique [2]

- The central limb is drawn along the distal ridge of the first webspace, extending from the proximal digital crease of the thumb to 1 cm proximal to the index digital crease at a point corresponding to the radial junction between the proximal and middle palmar crease (Fig. 2.1).
- Draw the proximal limb extending in a volar direction at a 90° or 120° angle to the proximal end of the central limb.
- The distal limb is directed dorsally relative to the central limb at an equal angle and length to the proximal palmar limb.
- Each angle is then bisected with another limb creating four equal flaps of 45° or 60° angle relative to the central limb.
- All limbs should be of equal length.

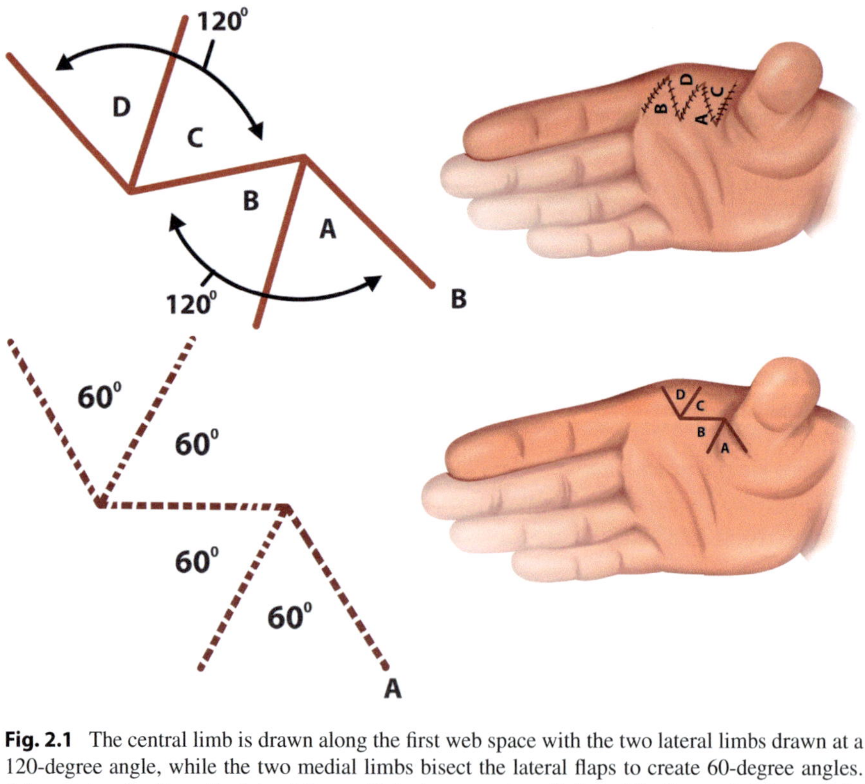

Fig. 2.1 The central limb is drawn along the first web space with the two lateral limbs drawn at a 120-degree angle, while the two medial limbs bisect the lateral flaps to create 60-degree angles. After raising the flaps, the lateral flaps will be transposed medially, while the medial flap will be transposed laterally (ABCD → CADB)

- Reversal of the proximal and distal limbs into proximal dorsal and distal palmer can be done if local condition necessitates (i.e., previous incision and specific approach for another concurrent procedure) with a satisfactory result; however, the former marking results in superior esthetic results as it parallels the interthenar crease.

Surgical Technique [2]
- After achieving proper anesthesia, the tourniquet is inflated.
- Skin incision is carried out along the marking.
- The flap is raised with careful undermining till the corresponding bases.
- If additional depth is needed, a small part of the underlying musculature is divided.
- Hemostasis is secured.
- The flaps are transposed as shown in Fig. 2.1: the previously shared border of the central flaps will be located against the proximal and distal incision sites, and the medial borders of the outer flaps will be adjacent to one another. The flap configuration of "ABCD" will be rearranged to "CADB" after transposition.
- Tension-free closure is done.
- Nonadherent gauze is used for dressing with gentle compressive dressing to keep the first webspace expanded.

Postop Care [2]
- Wound inspection is performed at 10–14 days postoperatively.
- Thermoplastic splint is applied following initial dressing change; then, active and passive range of motion (ROM) exercises are initiated.
- Thermoplastic splint is worn at all times except while performing ROM exercises.
- Gradual weaning of the splint is done over the next few weeks according to individual progress in physiotherapy.

Complications
The complications were similar to those of Z-plasty.

References

1. Hundeshagen G, Zapata-Sirvent R, Goverman J, Branski LK. Tissue rearrangements: the power of the Z-Plasty. Clin Plast Surg. 2017 Oct;44(4):805–12.
2. Wolfe SW, Pederson WC, Kozin SH. Green's operative hand surgery. 6th ed. London: Elsevier; 2021.
3. Woolf RM, Broadbent TR. The four-flap Z-plasty. Plast Reconstr Surg. 1972 Jan;49(1):48–51.
4. Rehim S, Chung K. Local flaps of the hand. Hand Clin. 2014;30(2):137–51.

Limberg (Rhomboid) Flap 3

Malak Alsaif and Mohammed Alfawzan

Classification [1] Random pattern local flap.

Vascular Supply Subdermal plexus.

Innervation N/A.

Indications [1–3]
- Small- to medium-sized defects in which the skin defect cannot be closed primarily as these flaps allow adequate tissue coverage with least donor site morbidity.

Contraindications
- Crush injuries
- Presence of active local infection
- Excessive scarring of the area.

Advantages [1, 2]
- Simple technique
- Primary closure of the donor area [1, 2]
- Less undermining
- Reconstructing the defect with like-for-like skin and color match.

M. Alsaif · M. Alfawzan (✉)
Plastic Surgery Division, Department of Surgery, Ministry of National Guard - Health Affairs, King Abdullah International Medical Research Center, Riyadh, Saudi Arabia

O. Almeshal et al. (eds.), *Soft Tissue Reconstruction of the Hand: Loco-regional and Distant Flaps Selection and Approach*,
https://doi.org/10.1007/978-981-16-9945-0_3

Disadvantages

- Requiring adequate adjacent healthy tissue
- Limited mobility and elasticity of hand skin
- Risk of necrosis if closed under tension.

Marking Technique [1, 4]

- The defect is converted into a rhomboid shape with two angles of 60 degrees and two angles of 120 degrees. Identical angles are opposing one another.
- After creating a rhomboid-shaped defect, we extend a line equal to the short access of the rhomboid (from the 120 degree angle). And the length of it, is equal to the length of the rhomboid.
- Another line is drawn from the end of the previous line and is parallel to either side of the rhomboid with a 60 degree angle (Fig. 3.1).

Surgical Technique [1, 2, 4]

- Under local anesthesia or general anesthesia, preparation and draping of the area in aseptic technique are done.
- After carefully designing the flap, a skin incision is performed over the marked area.
- The flap is elevated with adequate tissue undermining and transposed to cover the defect.
- The resultant secondary defect is then closed primarily.
- The line of closure of the secondary defect should be oriented in a way that does not result in excessive tension across the wound and to prevent puckering.

Postop Care

- General postop care includes flap monitoring for color, temperature, and capillary refill, hand elevation, analgesia, and regular dressing.

Complications

- Swelling/edema
- Infection
- Flap necrosis
- Hypertrophic scar/keloid
- Contractures.

Variants

- Dufourmentel flap [5, 6].

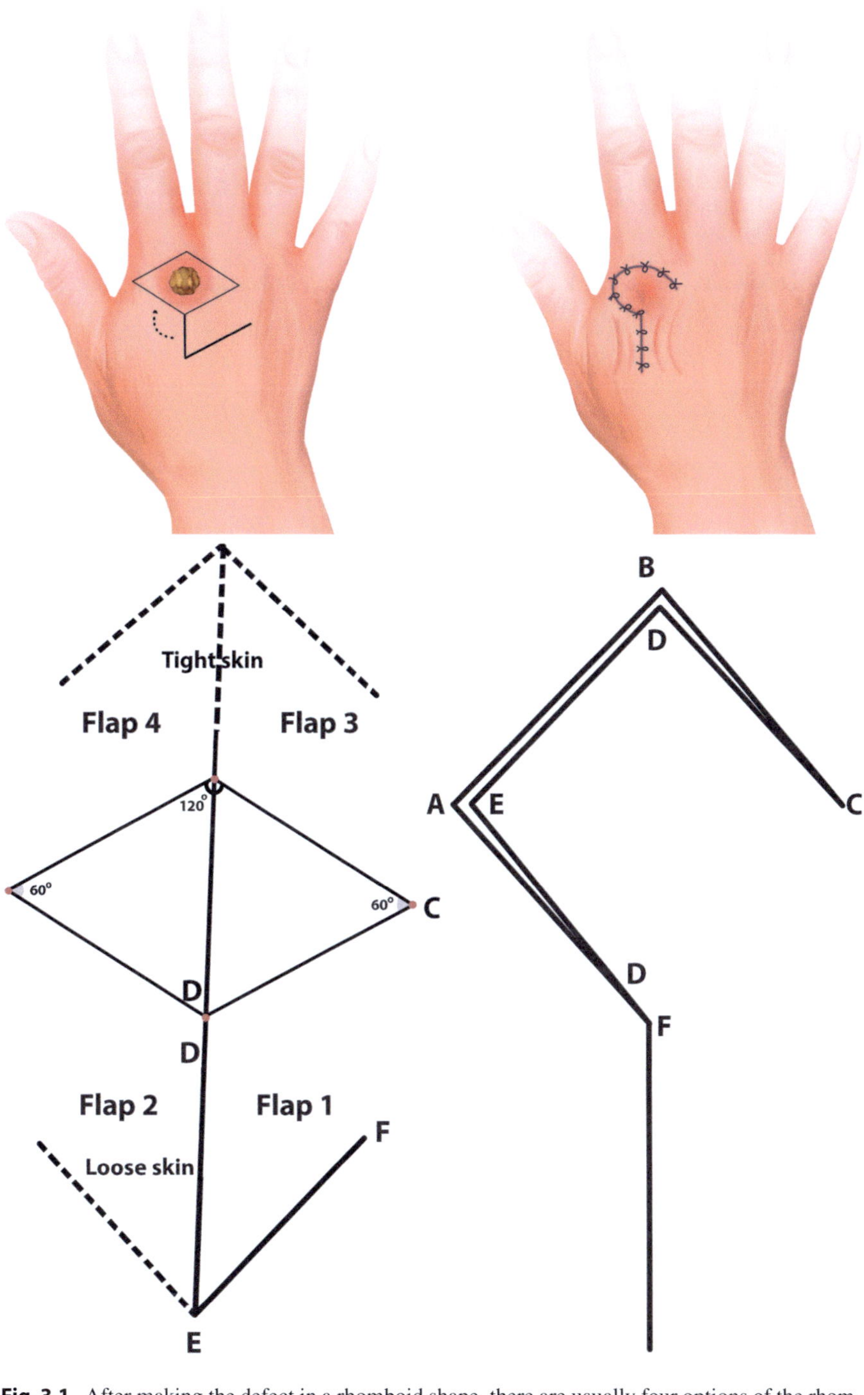

Fig. 3.1 After making the defect in a rhomboid shape, there are usually four options of the rhomboid flaps to be transposed by extending the short access of the defect and then drawing parallel lines to the long limbs of the defect. The flap choice depends on the mobility of the surrounding skin

References

1. Rehim SA, Chung KC. Local flaps of the hand. Hand Clin. 2014 May;30(2):137–51.
2. Hegge T, Henderson M, Amalfi A, Bueno RA, Neumeister MW. Scar contractures of the hand. Clin Plast Surg. 2011 Oct;38(4):591–606.
3. Chasmar LR. The versatile rhomboid (Limberg) flap. Can J Plast Surg. 2007 Summer;15(2):67–71.
4. Aydin OE, Tan O, Algan S, Kuduban SD, Cinal H, Barin EZ. Versatile use of rhomboid flaps for closure of skin defects. Eurasian J Med. 2011 Apr;43(1):1–8.
5. Limberg AA. Design of local flaps. Mod Trends Plast Surg. 1966;2:38–61.
6. Sebastian M, Sroczynski M, Rudnicki J. The Dufourmentel modification of the Limberg flap: does it fit all? Adv Clin Exp Med. 2017 Jan–Feb;26(1):63–7.

4 Rotational Flap

Malak Alsaif and Mohammed Alfawzan

Classification [1, 2] Random pattern local hand flap

The flap is rotated over a pivot point around which the tension of closure is distributed equally over a large surface area of the curved flap.

Vascular Supply Subdermal plexus.

Innervation N/A.

Indications [3]

- When primary closure of the skin could not be achieved
- When redirection of tension is indicated to prevent distortion
- Defects up to 3–5 cm, especially on the dorsum of the hand.

Contraindications

- Scar over proposed flap area
- Local radiotherapy that is believed to impair local vascular supply.

Advantages

- Simple technique
- Less undermining
- Reconstructing the defect with like-for-like skin and color match.

Disadvantages [2]

- Requiring adequate adjacent healthy tissue
- Limited mobility and elasticity of hand skin
- Probably needing a back cut, which might jeopardize the flap at the base.

M. Alsaif · M. Alfawzan (✉)
Plastic Surgery Division, Department of Surgery, Ministry of National Guard - Health Affairs, King Abdullah International Medical Research Center, Riyadh, Saudi Arabia

O. Almeshal et al. (eds.), *Soft Tissue Reconstruction of the Hand: Loco-regional and Distant Flaps Selection and Approach*,
https://doi.org/10.1007/978-981-16-9945-0_4

Marking Technique [1–3]

- The defect is outlined in a triangular fashion.
- The apex of the marked triangle represents the pivotal point around which the flap will be rotated and should be pointing toward the center of the flap, which is two to three times the length of the base of the flap.
- The base of the triangle is then extended to be continuous with the arc of the flap. The arc of rotation is designed to be five to eight times larger than the side of the triangle to permit adequate rotation of the flap without excessive tension.
- A back cut known as Burow's triangle can be added to gain extra length to rotate the flap. However, an excessive extension of the back cut will jeopardize the blood supply to the flap at the base and hence the viability of the flap (Fig. 4.1).

Surgical Technique [2, 4, 5]

- Rotation flaps are performed by creating a curvilinear incision.
- After completing the incision, a wide undermining is performed at the level of the subcutaneous plane, starting at the flap pivotal point.
- The flap is then rotated and transposed to the defect.
- Closure of the flap edges and donor is done without tension.

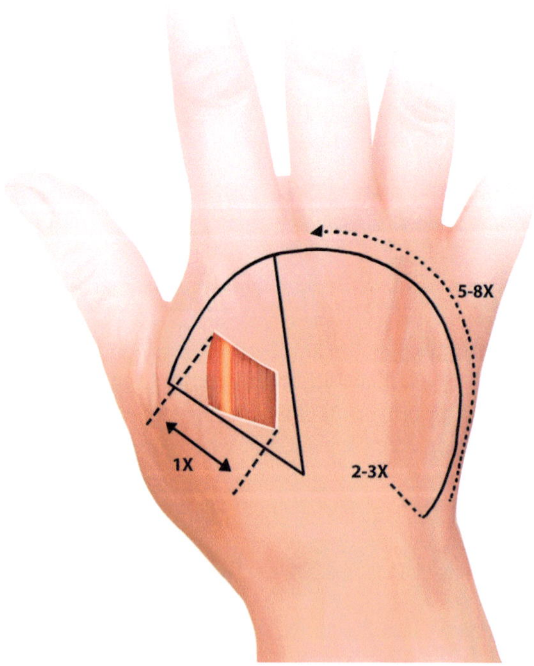

Fig. 4.1 The defect is triangulated with the apex of the triangle directed at the base of the pivot point. The limb's length is considered as "X." The arc of the rotational flap is drawn from the pivot point to the tip of the triangle with a length of "5–8 X." A back cut can be created to ease the mobility of the flap with a maximum length of "2–3 X"

Postop Care

- General postop care includes flap monitoring for color, temperature, and capillary refill, hand elevation, analgesia, and regular dressing.

Complications

- Swelling/edema
- Infection
- Flap necrosis
- Hypertrophic scar/keloid
- Contractures.

Variants

- Double rotation flaps
- O to Z flap.

Case

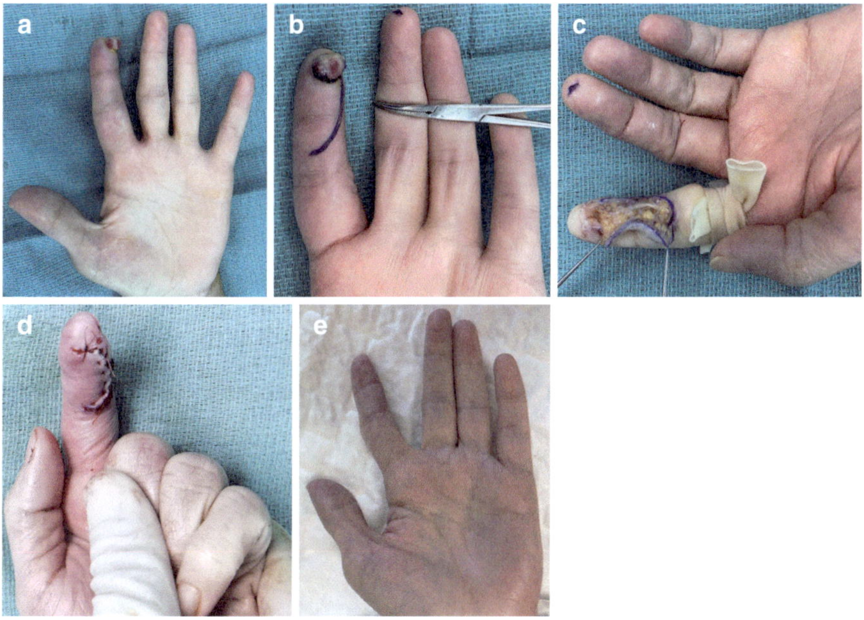

Case 4.1 Intraoperative photo of a patient who presented with pyogenic granuloma over the tip of the index finger in (**a**). In anticipation of the soft tissue defect, a rotation flap was marked over the volar side of the index finger distal and middle phalanx, as seen in (**b**). After excising the mass, the rotational flap was raised, as seen in (**c**). The flap was then rotated toward the defect and wounds were primarily closed as seen in (**d**). Follow-up assessment at two months showed good soft tissue coverage with a full range of motion as shown in (**e**)

References

1. Hurren JS, Cormack GC. The application of the rotation flap to the dorsum of the hand. Br J Plast Surg. 2000;53:491–4.
2. Rehim SA, Chung KC. Local Flaps of the hand. Hand Clin. 2014 May;30(2):137–51.
3. Maksoud A, Ahmed I. Rotation flap to cover a large defect on the dorsum of the hand. J Surg Case Rep. 2015 Nov;2015(11):139.
4. Kryger ZB, Sisco M. Practical plastic surgery. Austin, TX: Landes Bioscience; 2007. p. 43–55.
5. Lo CH, Kimble FW. The ideal rotation flap: an experimental study. J Plast Reconstr Aesthet Surg. 2008 Jul;61(7):754–9.

Bilobed Flap

5

Malak Alsaif and Mohammed Alfawzan

Classification [1, 2]
- Random pattern local flap
- Double transposition flap
- Originally described by Esser as 180-degree arc and then modified by Zitelli to 90-degree arc.

Vascular Supply Subdermal plexus.

Innervation N/A.

Indications [1]
- Used when other options on the reconstructive ladder fail to reconstruct the defect
- Used generally in areas where the skin is sparse and less mobile
- Large defects located on the dorsum of the hand, especially the thumb.

Contraindications [1, 2]
- Previous scars in the proposed flap site
- Relative contraindication in patients with suboptimal medical status such as smokers and patients who are taking anticoagulants.

Advantages
- Simple technique
- Less undermining
- Reconstructing the defect with like-for-like skin
- Color match.

M. Alsaif · M. Alfawzan (✉)
Plastic Surgery Division, Department of Surgery, Ministry of National Guard - Health Affairs, King Abdullah International Medical Research Center, Riyadh, Saudi Arabia

O. Almeshal et al. (eds.), *Soft Tissue Reconstruction of the Hand: Loco-regional and Distant Flaps Selection and Approach*,
https://doi.org/10.1007/978-981-16-9945-0_5

Disadvantages

- Requiring adequate adjacent healthy tissue
- Limited mobility and elasticity of hand skin
- Needing a secondary flap to close the resultant defect of the primary flap.

Marking Technique [1, 3–5]

- The defect is converted into a circle then triangulated.
- The center of the defect is marked and a line equal to the defect's radius is extended outside the defect into the proposed flap donor area. This point will be the pivot point of the primary lobe.
- A circle is now drawn around the marked pivot point and with a radius two times larger than that of the defect.
- A line is then drawn from the new pivot point in 45 degrees (A–C), which is equal in length to the A-B line, intersecting the circle.
- The point of intersection with the circle marks the edge of the primary lobe. The radius of the primary flap is equal to that of the defect (D–E equals E–F).
- Another line is extended from the pivot point in 90 degrees and the intersection point with the circle is marked; a secondary lobe is drawn with a radius equal to 2/3 to ½ of the radius of the defect (Fig. 5.1).
- An elliptical extension to the secondary lobe is then drawn. This extension allows reducing the chances of having a dog-ear deformity and allows for a more linear scar.

Surgical Technique

- Incision of the flap is made as per preoperative markings.
- The flaps are raised with wide undermining, ensuring uniformly equal thickness of the flap.
- The primary lobe is then transposed to the defect, with the secondary lobe transposed to the defect from the primary lobe.
- A deep absorbable suture was anchored at the angle between the two flaps, whereas the rest of the flaps were sutured in place.

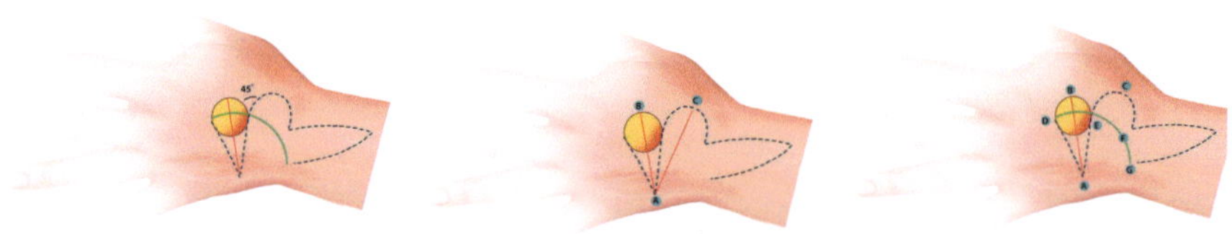

Fig. 5.1 After converting the defect into a circle, a triangular extension is made to the pivot point with a length equal to the radius of the circle. A–B line was bisecting the defect and considered as a reference point to the other flaps. A–C line drawn at 45 degrees from the A–B line to bisect the primary flap. The other flap is drawn with equal size of the defect. The second flap is drawn at 90 degrees from the pivot point with ½ of the size of the defect with elliptical extrusion to ease the closure

Postop Care

Postop care should be commenced while the patient is still in the operating room until after discharge. General postop care includes flap monitoring for color, temperature, and capillary refill, hand elevation, analgesia, and regular dressing.

Complications

- Swelling/edema
- Infection
- Flap necrosis.

Variants

- Zitelli bilobed flap [5].

Case

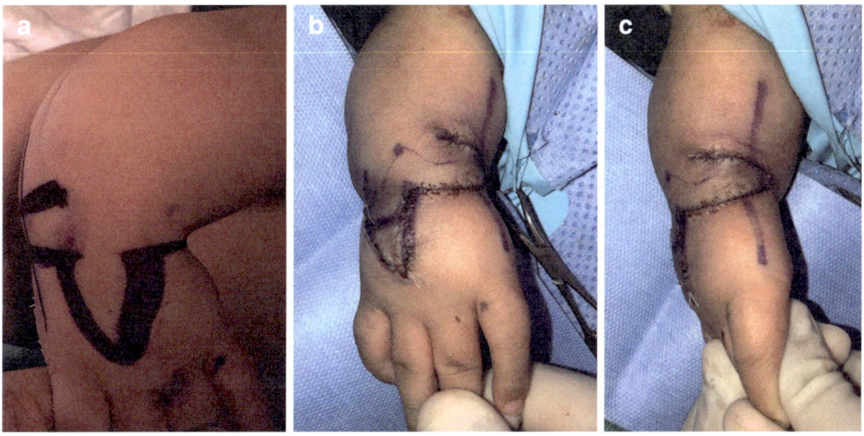

Case 5.1 Preoperative photo of a patient presented with radial club hand with expected skin deficiency after centralization procedure. In anticipation of the deficient skin coverage, the bilobed flap was marked over the dorsum of the wrist, as seen in (**a**). The flap was then raised from the ulnar and dorsal sides of the wrist and then transposed to cover the radial side of the wrist after the correction of the deformity, as seen in (**b**, **c**)

References

1. Agdoğan O, Karaçal R. Bilobed flap for reconstruction of a large keratoacanthoma of the thumb. Case Rep Plast Surg Hand Surg. 2019;6(1):86–7.
2. McGregor JC, Soutar DS. A critical assessment of the bilobed flap. Br J Plast Surg. 1981;34:197–205.
3. Miller CJ. Design principles for transposition flaps: the rhombic (single-lobed), bilobed, and trilobed flaps. Dermatol Surg. 2014;40:S43–52.
4. Nikkhah D, Jones M. The bilobed flap as a lifeboat flap for a forearm soft tissue defect. J Plast Reconstr Aesthet Surg. 2015 Aug;68(8):1153–4.
5. Zitelli JA. The bilobed flap for nasal reconstruction. Arch Dermatol. 1989 Jul;125:957–9.

V to Y Flap

6

Malak Alsaif and Mohammed Alfawzan

Classification [1] Random pattern local flap.

Vascular Supply Subdermal plexus.

Innervation N/A.

Indications [1–3]
- Incomplete congenital syndactyly with webbing proximal to PIP joint
- Hand contractures release:
  - Webspace contracture
  - Linear contracture with good skin cover
  - Dopuytren's contracture [4].

Contraindications [1]
Complete syndactyly with webbing distal to distal interphalangeal joint where more complex techniques and combination of techniques are indicated.

Advantages
- Simple flap design technique
- Short operative time
- Inconspicuous scar at the digital web
- Good match in skin color and texture.

M. Alsaif · M. Alfawzan (✉)
Plastic Surgery Division, Department of Surgery, Ministry of National Guard - Health Affairs, King Abdullah International Medical Research Center, Riyadh, Saudi Arabia

O. Almeshal et al. (eds.), *Soft Tissue Reconstruction of the Hand: Loco-regional and Distant Flaps Selection and Approach*,
https://doi.org/10.1007/978-981-16-9945-0_6

Disadvantages [5]

- It is limited to simple incomplete syndactyly.
- It cannot be used solely in complex or complete syndactyly.
- It might require an additional local flap to reconstruct the web [5].

Marking Technique [1, 5, 6]

- Syndactyly:
  - V-Y advancement flap is created by first marking a triangular flap on the affected webspace that is equal in size to the opposite unaffected mirror webspace on the contralateral hand.
  - After the triangular flap is marked, a straight line is extended proximally from the triangular apex to the level of the metacarpophalangeal (MCP) joint (Fig. 6.1).
- Contractures
  - The V-shaped flap is marked proximal to the contracture or scar
  - In certain cases, the V limbs are marked over the scar, such as Dupuytren's contracture [4].
  - Make sure that the skin in the transverse plane can be approximated for closure of the Y part of the flap.

Surgical Technique

- After completing the marking of the flap, a full-thickness skin incision is made with minimal undermining. Then, the triangular flap is transposed proximally to the level of the new webspace or advanced to release the tension over the contracted area, in a V-Y advancement style and is sutured in place.

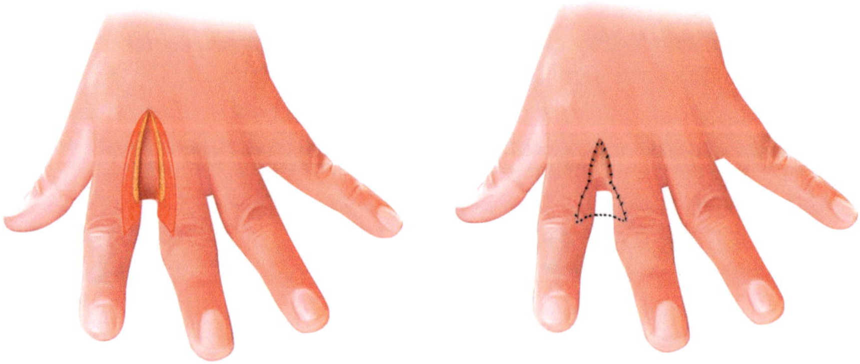

Fig. 6.1 The area is marked in V fashion, with the vertical limb being at the volar aspect of the webspace. The triangular flap is raised and it is advanced all the way to the vertical limb to create the webspace

Postop Care
General postop care includes flap monitoring, hand elevation, analgesia, and regular dressing.

Complications [2, 7]
- Hematoma/seroma
- Infection [7]
- Contractures
- Flap necrosis.

Variants
- V-M flap
- Three-flap web-plasty [8].

References

1. Yamashita K, Yotsuyanagi T, Yamauchi SMA, Gonda A, Shinji K, Kita A. Subcutaneous pedicle V-Y flap for release of incomplete congenital syndactyly. Plast Reconstr Aesthet Surg. 2016 Aug;69(8):86–91.
2. Karjalainen T, Sebastin SJ, Chee KG, Peng YP, Chong AKS. Flap related complications requiring secondary surgery in a series of 851 local flaps used for fingertip reconstruction. J Hand Surg Asian Pac. 2019 Mar;24(1):24–9.
3. Savaci N, Hosnuter M, Tosun Z. Use of reverse triangular V-Y flaps to create a web space in syndactyly. Ann Plast Surg. 1999;42:540–4.
4. Mahaffey PJ. V-Y plasty for Dupuytren's contracture of the palm. J R Coll Surg Edinb. 1996 Dec;41(6):425.
5. Yildirim C, Şentürk S, Keklikçi K, Akmaz I. Correction of syndactyly using a dorsal separated V-Y advancement flap and a volar triangular flap in adults. Ann Plast Surg. 2011 Aug;67(4):357–63.
6. Sherif MM. V-Y dorsal metacarpal flap: a new technique for the correction of syndactyly without skin graft. Plast Reconstr Surg. 1998;101:1861–6.
7. Karamese M, Akdag O, Selimoglu MN, Yıldıran GU, Tosun Z. V-Y and rectangular flap combination for syndactyly repair. J Plast Surg Hand Surg. 2016;50:102–6.
8. Ostrowski DM, Feagin CA, Gould JS. A three-flap web-plasty for release of short congenital syndactyly and dorsal adduction contracture. J Hand Surg Am. 1991 Jul;16(4):634–41.

V to M Flap

7

Malak Alsaif and Mohammed Alfawzan

Classification [1] V-M advancement flap is a random pattern local hand flap.

Vascular Supply Subdermal plexus.

Innervation N/A.

Indications
- Congenital complete or incomplete syndactyly
- Contractures
  - Acquired webspace contractures
  - Hand Scars and contractures release.

Contraindications
- Complex web loss and/or complex syndactyly requiring further reconstructive techniques rather than random pattern local flaps.

Advantages [1, 2]
- Versatility
- Preserving the normal contour of the affected web
- Allowing raising flap on a scarred tissue
- No need for a skin graft to close a secondary defect
- Minimal recurrence rate
- Short operative time
- Minimal blood loss
- Good match in skin color and texture.

M. Alsaif · M. Alfawzan (✉)
Plastic Surgery Division, Department of Surgery, Ministry of National Guard - Health Affairs, King Abdullah International Medical Research Center, Riyadh, Saudi Arabia

O. Almeshal et al. (eds.), *Soft Tissue Reconstruction of the Hand: Loco-regional and Distant Flaps Selection and Approach*,
https://doi.org/10.1007/978-981-16-9945-0_7

Disadvantages [1, 2]
- Limited to simple incomplete syndactyly
- Limited application to minor web contractures
- Probably requiring an additional local flap to reconstruct the web.

Marking Technique [1–3]
- Three triangular flaps are marked to execute this technique, each with an apex angle of around 60 degrees.
- First, a dorsal V-shaped flap is designed with an apex pointing into the affected web (Fig. 7.1).
- The other remaining two triangular flaps are designed adjacent to each other, which constitute the M flap on the volar aspect of the affected web.
- The bases of all triangular flaps should be marked at the level of the metacarpal bone head dorsally and volarly. The length of the triangular flap is determined by the distance between the metacarpal head at the furthest distal point of the fused/contracture digits, whereas the width of the flap is determined by the mid-dorsal and midvolar distance between the digits.

Surgical Technique [3]
- The operation is performed after ensuring adequate anesthesia and securing adequate hemostasis under the control of a pneumatic tourniquet.
- Perpendicular incisions over the marked flap lines are made.
- The flaps are then elevated on a subcutaneous plane.
- The dorsal V-shaped flap is then advanced to the web to intermingle the two volar flaps in a V-M manner.
- The two volar flaps are advanced to adjacent fingers wounds.
- Then, the surgical lines are closed primarily.

Postop Care
- General postop care includes flap monitoring for color, temperature, and capillary refill, hand elevation, and analgesia and regular dressing.

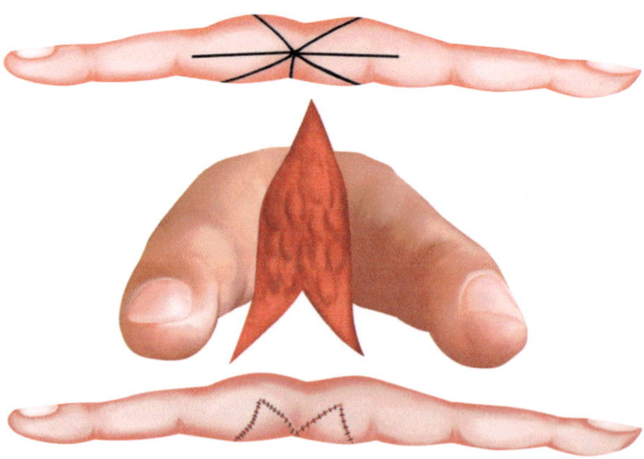

Fig. 7.1 Three triangular flaps are drawn, one in the dorsal aspect of the webspace with the apex designed toward the webspace, while the other two flaps are drawn on the volar aspect of the webspace. The flaps are raised in the usual fashion, then transposed to deepen the webspace with the dorsal flap advanced volarly and the two volar flaps laterally to each digit

Complications [2–4]

- Hematoma/seroma
- Infection
- Contractures
- Flap necrosis (tip of triangular necrosis).

Variants

- Z-plasty
- V-N plasty [5]
- Opposing V-Y-Z plasty [6]
- Modified Cronin method (inverted V-shaped flaps) [7].

References

1. Tan O, Atik B, Ergen D. Versatile use of the VM-plasty for reconstruction of the web space. Ann Plast Surg. 2005;55:623–8.
2. Davami B. V-M plasty and double Z-plasty two versatile flaps for treatment of postburn syndactyly. Tech Hand Surg. 2009;13:124–9.
3. Alexander JW, MacMillan BG, Martel L. Correction of post-burn syndactyly: an analysis of children with introduction of the VM-plasty and postoperative pressure inserts. Plast Reconstr Surg. 1982;70:345–52.
4. Gulgonen A, Ozer K. The correction of postburn contractures of the second through fourth web spaces. J Hand Surg. 2007;32:556–64.
5. Kollali EL, R, Ghoneim I, Azemi MA. V-N plasty for the release of severe postburn contractures. J Plast Reconstr Surg. 2006;59:1424–8.
6. Tan O, Atik B, Ergen D. A new method in the treatment of postburn scar contractures: double opposing V-Y-Z plasty. Burns. 2006;32:499–503.
7. Cronin TD. Syndactylism: results of zigzag incision to prevent postoperative contracture. Plast Reconstr Surg. 1956;18:460–8.

Simple Transposition Flap

8

Malak Alsaif and Mohammed Alfawzan

Classification [1, 2] Random pattern local hand flap.

Vascular Supply Subdermal plexus.

Innervation N/A.

Indications [1, 2]
- When simpler options in the reconstructive ladder result in less appealing results
- When reconstruction with simpler techniques in the reconstructive ladder poses a risk of suboptimal function
- When size and location permit simpler local manipulation of tissues

Contraindications [1]
- Crush injuries
- Local wound infections
- Local radiation and scarring

Advantages [2]
- Simple technique
- Less undermining
- Reconstructing the defect with like-for-like skin and color match

Disadvantages [2]
- Requiring adequate adjacent healthy tissue
- Limited mobility and elasticity of hand skin

M. Alsaif · M. Alfawzan (✉)
Plastic Surgery Division, Department of Surgery, Ministry of National Guard - Health Affairs, King Abdullah International Medical Research Center, Riyadh, Saudi Arabia

O. Almeshal et al. (eds.), *Soft Tissue Reconstruction of the Hand: Loco-regional and Distant Flaps Selection and Approach*,
https://doi.org/10.1007/978-981-16-9945-0_8

Marking Technique

- The defect is triangulated into an isosceles triangle and the apex of the triangle is preferably designed to be narrow as that will allow minimal advancement of the flap (Fig. 8.1).
- The transposition flap is designed to be in contact with the triangulated defect in a rectangular fashion.
- For marking the flap, a line equal to the height of one side of the isosceles is drawn from the apex (YX).

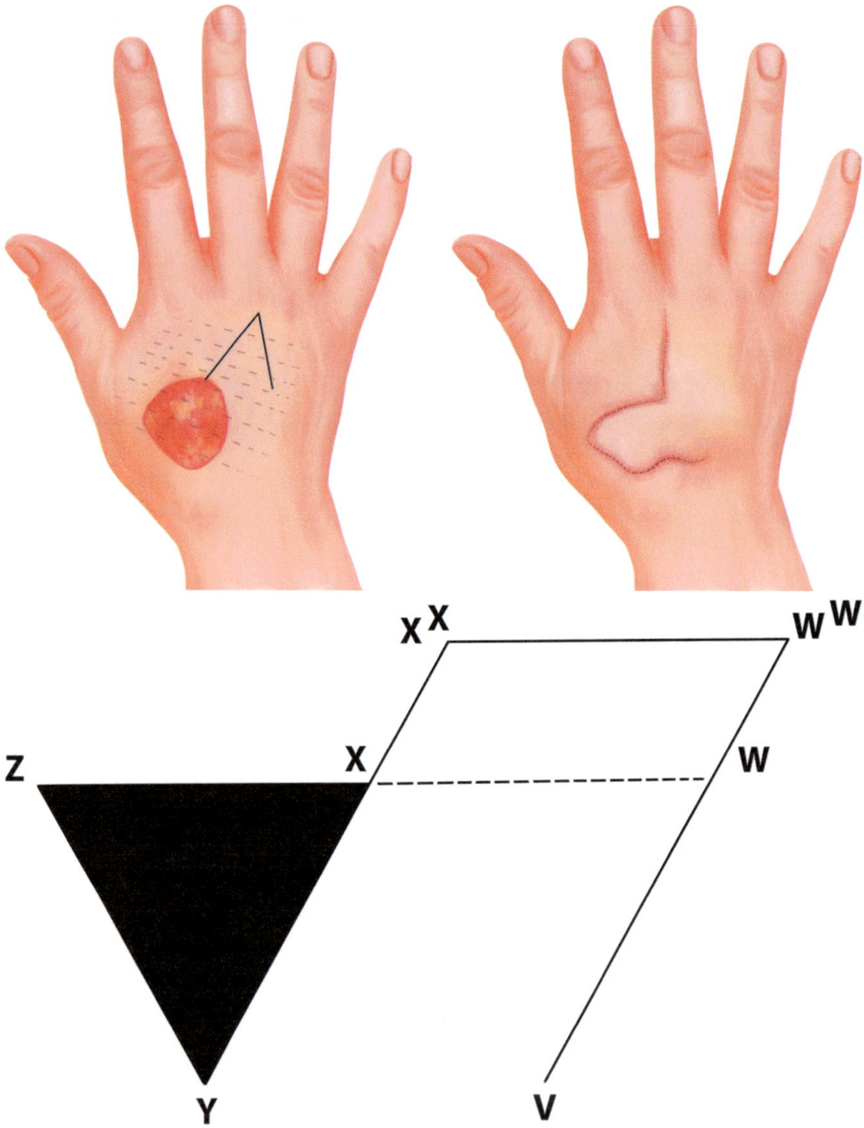

Fig. 8.1 The defect is triangulated to equal limbs to minimize the tension of the transposition. The advancing limb of the flap is the one adjacent to the defect (YX). The other limb is drawn parallel to its line (VW) with a distance usually larger than the defect to transpose it easily from the pivot point

- Then, a line arbitrarily extended from one side of the isosceles triangle (XW) and another parallel line from the pivot point (WV) are drawn.
- The flap should be larger in height than that of the original defect so that it can close the defect ideally.
- A line of maximal tension extended from the pivot point to the opposite angle of the isosceles is measured and rotated until it intersected with the arbitrary lines. These points of intersection mark the superior side of the flap.

Surgical Technique [2, 3]
- After marking is done, the flap is elevated with subcutaneous plane undermining.
- The flap is advanced over the pivot point to close the defect.
- A resultant dog-ear deformity might present, which can then be excised and closed primarily.
- In classic transposition flaps, a secondary defect might result, which mandates a closure with a skin graft.

Postop Care
- General postop care includes flap monitoring for color, temperature and capillary refill, hand elevation, and analgesia and regular dressing

Complications [4, 5]
- Swelling/edema
- Infection
- Flap necrosis
- Hypertrophic scar/keloid

Variants
- Limberg rhomboid flaps
- Bilobed flap

Case

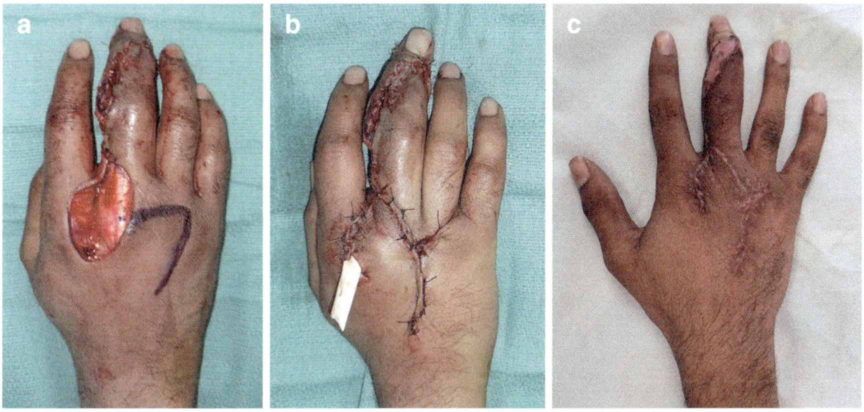

Case 8.1 Intraoperative photo of a patient presented with soft tissue defect over the hand dorsum as a secondary wound after raising an inter-commissural flap to cover middle finger defect. Coverage was planned with random transposition flap marked over the remaining hand dorsal skin as seen in (**a**). Flap was raised and then transposed over the defect and the wounds were primarily closed as seen in (**b**). Follow-up assessment at two months showed intact soft tissue coverage as seen in (**c**)

References

1. Rehim SA, Chung KC. Local flaps of the hand. Hand Clin. 2014 May;30(2):137–51.
2. Lister G. The theory of the transposition flap and its practical application in the hand. Clin Plast Surg. 1981 Jan;8(1):115–27.
3. Starkman SJ, Williams CT, Sherris DA. Flap basics I: rotation and transposition flaps. Facial Plast Surg Clin North Am. 2017 Aug;25(3):313–21.
4. Vartanian E, Gould DJ, Lee SW, Patel KM. Pilonidal disease: classic and contemporary concepts for surgical management. Ann Plast Surg. 2018 Dec;81(6):12–9.
5. Molenkamp S, Waterbolk TW, Mariani MA, Werker PM. Predictors of complications after pectoralis major transposition for sternum dehiscence. Ann Plast Surg. 2017 Feb;78(2):208–12.

Part II

Finger tip Flaps: V-Y Advancement Flaps

(Atasoy) Flap

9

Muhammad Majid Ul Haq and Mohammed Alfawzan

The first description of a triangular flap designed for fingertip pulp defects was by Tranquilli-Leali in 1935. However, it was popularized by Atasoy and his colleagues in 1970 [1].

Classification [1]

- Random pattern flap
- Flap dimensions from 10 to 15 mm
- Advancement up to 10 mm

Vascular Supply [1]

- Vascular supply is ensured from terminal branches of digital arteries:
  - Pulp anastomotic arch
  - Palmar digital artery
  - Flexor tendon
  - Pulp-destined terminal branch
  - Central artery of the pulp

Indications [1]

Atasoy flap is mainly indicated for transverse or dorsal oblique fingertip amputations.

Contraindications

- Volar oblique amputations

M. M. Ul Haq · M. Alfawzan (✉)
Plastic Surgery Division, Department of Surgery, Ministry of National Guard - Health Affairs, King Abdullah International Medical Research Center, Riyadh, Saudi Arabia

O. Almeshal et al. (eds.), *Soft Tissue Reconstruction of the Hand: Loco-regional and Distant Flaps Selection and Approach*,
https://doi.org/10.1007/978-981-16-9945-0_9

Advantages

- Simple and reliable dissection
- Sensate skin
- Primary closure of the donor

Disadvantages

- Little advancement only
- Contour distortion of the fingertip
- Hook nail deformity

Marking Technique [2, 3]

- A triangle shape is drawn (letter V), with its base adjacent to the defect and apex at the distal interphalangeal crease (Fig. 9.1).
- The flap edges should be at least 1.5 times the planned advancement.
- The V angle should be at least 30 to decrease the chances of ischemia.

Surgical Technique [2, 3]

- Local anesthesia is applied or digital block if the patient is reliable. Otherwise, general anesthesia is recommended.
- Thorough debridement of the wound is done, including shortening of the bone, followed by irrigation.

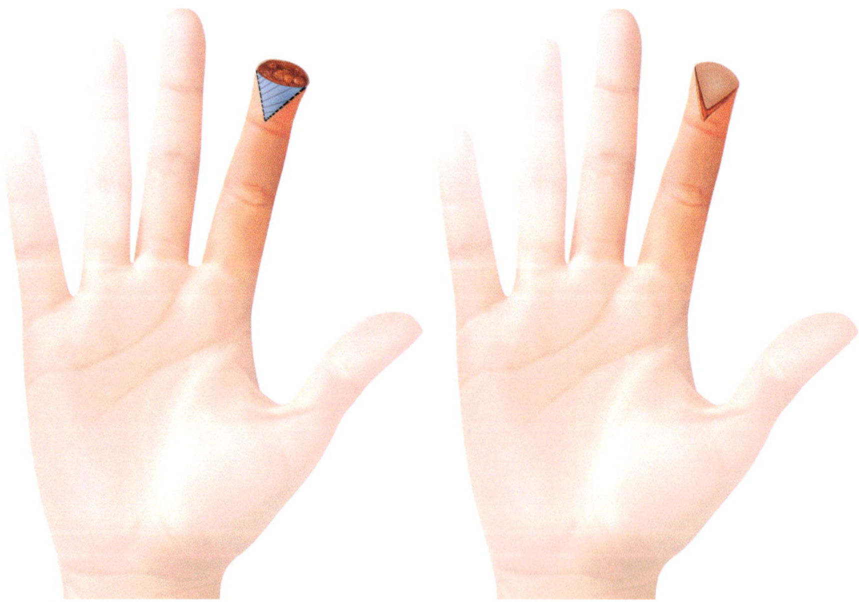

Fig. 9.1 The flap is designed with the apex at the DIP crease, and the leading edge of the flap is the defect. The incision is made to the subcutaneous tissue only; then, the flap is released from the periosteum to advance it easily, and it is closed in a V-Y fashion

- After marking, only the skin of the lateral flap edges is incised and no incision is made in the subcutaneous tissue.
- For advancement, the deep surface of the flap must be completely released from the periosteum of the underlying phalanx, using a scalpel, making every effort to stay close to the bone.
- Laterally, the fibrous bands that restrict the mobility of the skin island are released.
- Elevation and advancement of the flap are done, and suturing usually starts distally at flap borders and then at the donor site into a "V-Y" configuration.
- If the flap is compromised after suturing, release of sutures is done to relieve tension.

Postop Care
- Dressing with sterile petroleum-soaked gauze and bandage
- Antibiotics course for 3 days
- Early mobilization of finger PIP and MCP joints

Complications
- A shortened distal phalanx results in the loss of nail bed support.
- A hook nail deformity can occur. (Excision of the sterile nail matrix 2 mm proximal to the shortened bone can help prevent this complication.) The patient is taught to trim the nail frequently.
- A V-Y advancement flap creates additional incisions over the volar finger pulp. Hypertrophic and hypersensitive scarring can occur.

Variants
- It is worth mentioning that, in the original description, full-thickness incisions were made down to the periosteum, with no subperiosteal elevation, keeping the flap attached to the underlying bone.
- The flap is not sutured for better vascularity and contour of the pulp; instead, a K-wire is inserted through the flap to the distal phalanx to secure the flap, leaving the donor and wound edges to heal by secondary intention.
- "V-Y cup flap," the two edges of the base of the flap are sutured together to form a cup.

Case

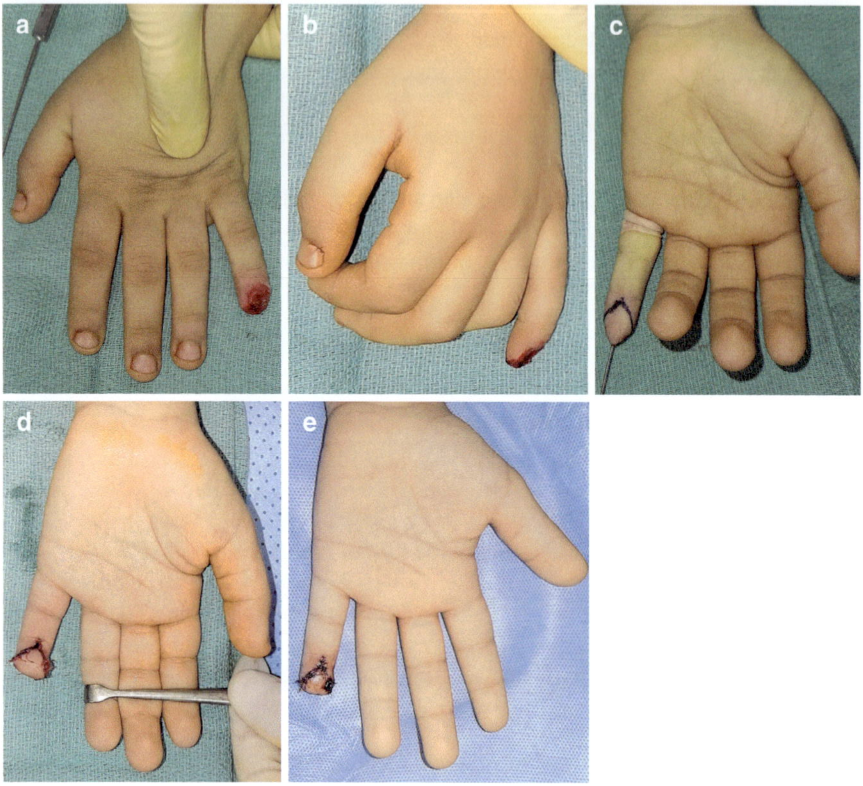

Case 9.1 Intraoperative photo of a patient who presented with dorsal oblique fingertip injury with soft tissue loss in (**a**, **b**). The wound was irrigated and cleaned; after that, coverage was planned with a volar V-Y (Atasoy) advancement flap marked over the pulp of the distal phalanx, as seen in (**c**). The flap was then raised and advanced to cover the defect, as seen in (**d**). Follow-up assessment at 3 weeks showed good soft tissue coverage, as seen in (**e**)

References

1. Atasoy E, Igakimidis E, Kaspak ML, Kutz JE, Kleinert HC. Reconstruction of the amputated fingertip with a triangular volar flap: a new surgical procedure. J Bone Joint Surg. 1970;52A:921–6.
2. Lim JX, Chung KC. VY advancement, thenar flap, and cross-finger flaps. Hand Clin. 2020 Feb;36(1):19–32.
3. Foo TL, Wan KH, Chew WY. Safe and easy method to preserve fingertip contour in VY-plasty. Tech Hand Up Extrem Surg. 2012 Jun;16(2):95–7.

Bilateral V-Y (Kutler) Flap

10

Muhammad Majid Ul Haq and Mohammed Alfawzan

The bilateral flap was introduced in 1937. Its principle is similar to that of Atasoy; it involves the advancement of skin triangles on a hinge of the subcutaneous pulp tissue [1, 2].

Classification

- Random pattern flap

Vascular Supply [3, 4]

- Vascular supply is ensured from terminal branches of digital arteries:
  - Pulp anastomotic arch
  - Palmar digital artery
  - Flexor tendon
  - Pulp-destined terminal branch
  - Central artery of the pulp

Innervation

Digital neurovascular bundle branches (abundant on the palmar aspect of the finger and sparse on the lateral and dorsal areas)

Indications

- Short beveled palmar or low oblique amputations in area
- Palmar oblique or asymmetrical fingertip amputation

M. M. Ul Haq · M. Alfawzan (✉)
Plastic Surgery Division, Department of Surgery, Ministry of National Guard - Health Affairs, King Abdullah International Medical Research Center, Riyadh, Saudi Arabia

O. Almeshal et al. (eds.), *Soft Tissue Reconstruction of the Hand: Loco-regional and Distant Flaps Selection and Approach*,
https://doi.org/10.1007/978-981-16-9945-0_10

Contraindication

- The obliqueness of the amputation that reduces the effective area of residual proximal pulp and makes it difficult to use

Advantages [4, 5]

- Simple and reliable dissection
- Sensate skin
- Primary closure of donor

Disadvantages

- Limited advancement
- Hypersensitivity or numbness
- Hook nail deformity

Marking Technique [6, 7]

- The triangles are centered at the mid-lateral line.
- Base is at the wound's edge.
- The apex is at the distal interphalangeal crease (Fig. 10.1)

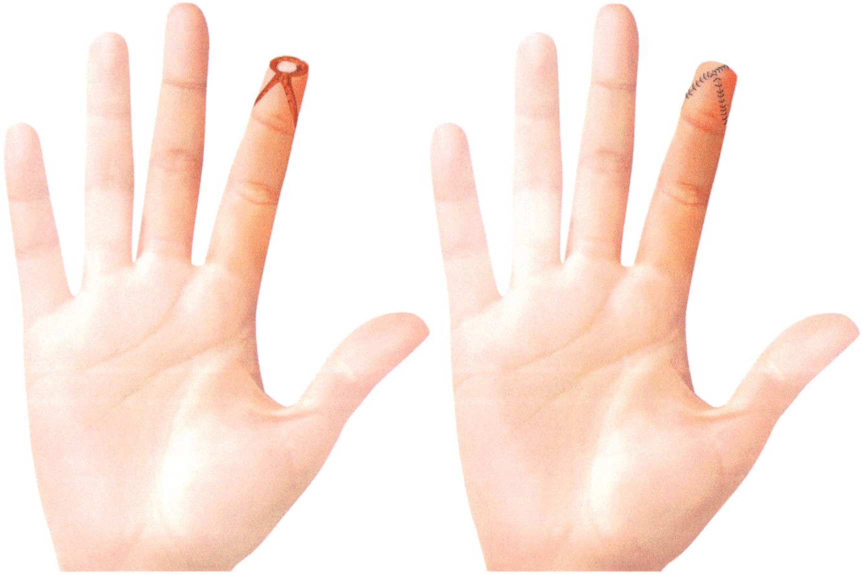

Fig. 10.1 In a similar fashion to Atasoy V-Y, two triangular flaps are designed centered along the midaxillary line. The incision is only to the skin down to the subcutaneous tissue. The fibrous septa from the underlying periosteum to ease flap advancement to the midline are released, and the two flaps are sutured together

Surgical Technique [6, 7]

- Local anesthesia is applied or digital block if the patient is reliable. Otherwise, general anesthesia is recommended.
- Thorough debridement of the wound is done, including shortening of the bone, followed by irrigation.
- The two flaps are matched at the midline.
- The skin is incised without violating the subcutaneous tissue.
- The fibrous septa from the periosteum are released.
- Then, the flap is medially pulled with a Gillies hook; the remaining septa are released.
- Advancement is made on a hinge of the subcutaneous pulp tissue.
- The flap is fixated to the contralateral flap with sutures.
- The donor is closed in a “Y” form bilaterally.
- Advancement up to 4 mm is done.

Postop Care [7]

- The postop care protocol is the same as that of Atasoy flap

Complications

- Due to the flaps’ small size and little advancement, it has very limited clinical value.
- They also result in a midline scar on the pulp, which may become problematic.

Variants

- In 1976, Segmüller modified this flap by dissecting the neurovascular pedicle at the base of the tip of the skin triangle, turning it into an island flap [1, 3].
- The apex of the flaps is extended to the proximal interphalangeal crease, given a higher risk of complications.

Case

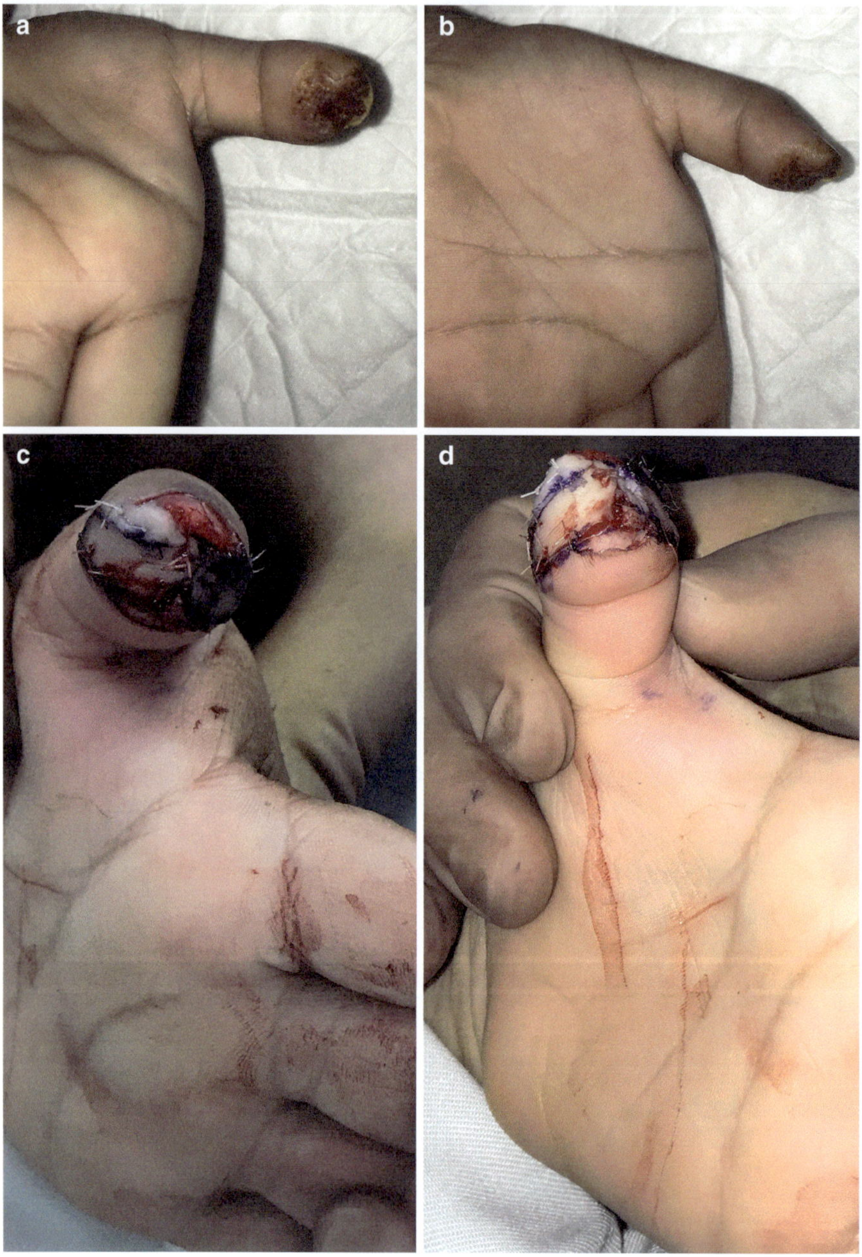

Case 10.1 Preoperative photo of a patient who presented with a chronic wound over the pulp of the distal phalanx of the thumb in (**a**, **b**). After debridement, coverage of the remaining exposed wound was planned with bilateral V-Y advancement flaps. The flaps were marked and elevated and then advanced over the defect, ensuring good soft tissue coverage as seen in (**c**, **d**)

References

1. Lim JX, Chung KC. VY advancement, thenar flap, and cross-finger flaps. Hand Clin. 2020 Feb;36(1):19–32.
2. Kutler W. A new method for fingertip amputation. JAMA. 1947;133:29–30.
3. Segmuller G. Modification des Kutler-Lappens neurovaskuläre stielung. Handchir. 1976;8:75–6.
4. Gharb BB, Rampazzo A, Armijo BS, Eshraghi Y, Totonchi AS, Teo TC, Salgado CJ. Tranquilli-Leali or Atasoy flap: an anatomical cadaveric study. J Plast Reconstr Aesthet Surg. 2010 Apr;63(4):681–5.
5. Foo TL, Wan KH. Modification of VY flap to preserve fingertip contour. Hand (N Y). 2012 Dec;7(4):388–90.
6. Foo TL, Wan KH, Chew WY. Safe and easy method to preserve fingertip contour in VY-plasty. Tech Hand Up Extrem Surg. 2012 Jun;16(2):95–7.
7. Wolfe S. Green's operative hand surgery. 7th ed. New York: Elsevier; 2004.

Oblique Triangular (Venkataswami) Flap 11

Hazqeel Solangi and Mohammed Alfawzan

Classification [1] Axial pattern flap based on known digital artery

Vascular Supply Digital artery

Innervation Digital nerve

Indications
- Volar and dorsal oblique fingertip amputation
- Transverse defects and oblique defects in the lateral aspect at zone I or II

Contraindications
- Prior injury of the digital vessels
- History of angiopathy affecting the vessels of the hand, such as vasospasm, vasculitis, peripheral vascular disease, or embolism
- Large defects >2 cm

Advantages
- Well-padded glabrous skin
- Sensate skin
- Avoiding midline scar formation in the fingertip

Disadvantages
- Relatively complex dissection
- Medial limb longitudinal scar that can predispose to scar contracture

H. Solangi · M. Alfawzan (✉)
Plastic Surgery Division, Department of Surgery, Ministry of National Guard - Health Affairs, King Abdullah International Medical Research Center, Riyadh, Saudi Arabia

O. Almeshal et al. (eds.), *Soft Tissue Reconstruction of the Hand: Loco-regional and Distant Flaps Selection and Approach*,
https://doi.org/10.1007/978-981-16-9945-0_11

Marking Technique [2]

- The flap is outlined beginning at the mid-lateral line and is extended proximally 2.5 times the diameter of the wound (Fig. 11.1).
- The flap design is oblique triangular V-shaped.
- The base of the triangle lies adjacent to the wound.
- The apex of the triangle is marked at the PIP joint.
- Vertical (dorsal) limb is lying in the mid-lateral line.
- Oblique (volar) limb is pointed from the downward margin of the base to join the apex.

Surgical Technique [2]

- The surgery is conducted under general or regional anesthesia.
- Tourniquet control with sterile paint and drapes is utilized.
- After flap markings, the vertical incision is made in the mid-lateral line of the finger down to the periosteum (care is taken to preserve the neurovascular bundle), and the pedicle is fully raised, avoiding skeletonization.
- Then, partial-thickness oblique incision is made, and only the fibrous septa are divided to allow flap advancement.
- After elevation, the flap is advanced, inset, and then closed in a V-Y fashion.
- The donor site is usually closed primarily.
- Advancing the flap while PIP and DIP joint are in extension (rather than flexing the joints while advancing) may decrease flexion contracture.
- This technique can offer up to 15 mm advancement.

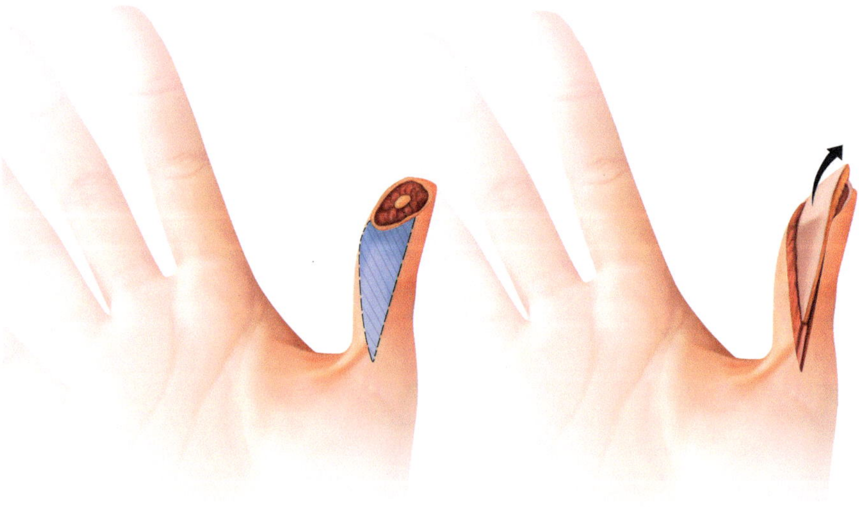

Fig. 11.1 The flap is designed obliquely to include one neurovascular bundle in it. It can be extended down to PIP joint. The first incision is made along the mid-axial line dorsal to the bundle down to the periosteum, while the other oblique incision is made to the subcutaneous tissue. The flap is advanced by releasing the fibrous attachment to close the defect

Postop Care

- Local wound care
- Initiation of ROM exercises soon after wound healing to prevent finger joint stiffness

Complications [3, 4]

- Sensory disturbance, especially if advancement was more than 12 mm
- PIP joint flexion contracture
- Partial flap necrosis or total flap necrosis

Variants [2]

- In 1988, Evans and Martin modified this technique:
  - The flap design was modified by creating a step pattern along the medial incision instead of the traditional straight line.
  - The advantage of this modification is that it minimizes the risk of scar contracture and retraction of skin paddle.

Case

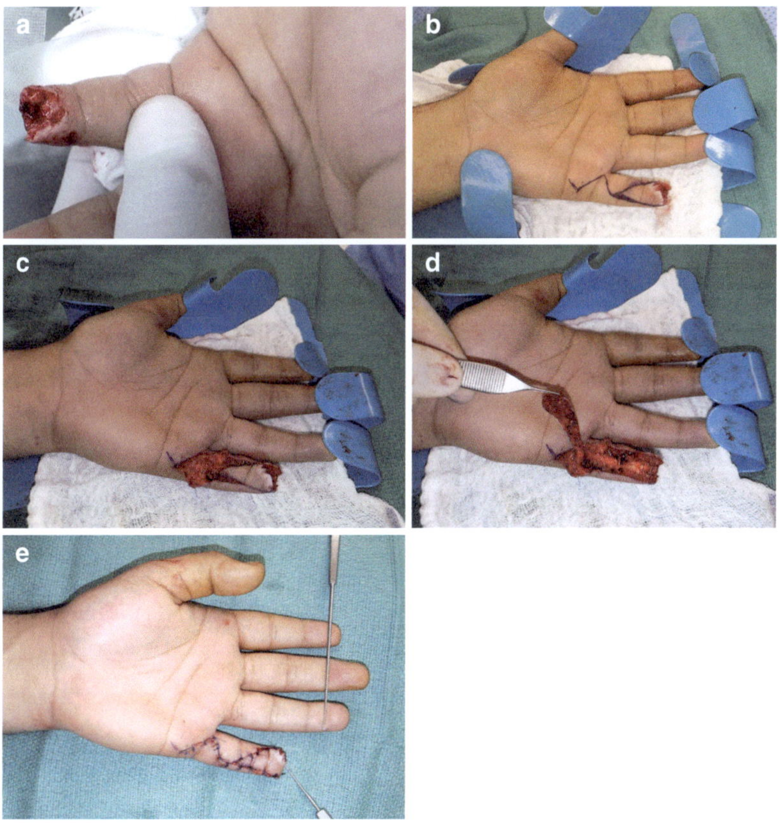

Case 11.1 Preoperative photo of a patient who presented with traumatic amputation of little finger distal phalanx with exposed bone in (**a**). Soft tissue coverage was planned with oblique triangular (Venkataswami) flap that was marked over the remaining distal and middle phalanx volar till mid-lateral line as seen in (**b**). The flap was then raised with its pedicle based on the digital neurovascular bundle as seen in (**c**, **d**). The flap was then advanced and inset to cover the defect as seen in (**e**)

References

1. Venkataswami DR, Subramanian N. Oblique triangular flap: a new method of repair for oblique amputations of the fingertip and thumb. Plast Reconstr Surg. 1980;66:296–300.
2. Evans DM, Martin DL. Step-advancement island flap for fingertip reconstruction. Br J Plast Surg. 1988;41(2):105–11.
3. Sano K, Ozeki S, Kimura K, Hyakusoku H. Relationship between sensory recovery and advancement distance of oblique triangular flap for fingertip reconstruction. J Hand Surg Am. 2008 Sep;33(7):1088–92.
4. Usami S, Kawahara S, Yamaguchi Y, Hirase T. Homodigital artery flap reconstruction for fingertip amputation: a comparative study of the oblique triangular neurovascular advancement flap and the reverse digital artery island flap. J Hand Surg Eur. 2015 Mar;40(3):291–7.

Segmüller Flap

12

Maher Elnahas and Mohammed Alfawzan

Segmüller [1] described a variant of the Kutler flap that is raised as an island on its neurovascular bundle and has a much bigger volume and mobility than the Kutler flap. Originally, the flap was raised only proximally as far as the DIP joint crease.

Classification [2–5] Pedicled V-Y advancement island flap, unilateral or bilateral

Vascular Supply [4, 5] Ipsilateral digital artery

Innervation [4, 5] Ipsilateral digital nerve.

Indications [3–5]
- Volar "palmar" oblique amputation
- Transverse amputation at the proximal third of the nail plate

Contraindications [3, 6]
- Prior injury of the digital vessels
- History of angiopathy affecting the vessels of the hand, such as vasospasm, vasculitis, peripheral vascular disease, or embolism
- Large defects >2 cm

Advantages [3, 4, 7]
- A single-stage reconstruction
- Good flap advancement and cover potential (up to 20 mm)
- Sensate flap

M. Elnahas · M. Alfawzan (✉)
Plastic Surgery Division, Department of Surgery, Ministry of National Guard - Health Affairs, King Abdullah International Medical Research Center, Riyadh, Saudi Arabia

O. Almeshal et al. (eds.), *Soft Tissue Reconstruction of the Hand: Loco-regional and Distant Flaps Selection and Approach*,
https://doi.org/10.1007/978-981-16-9945-0_12

- Good padding and contour of the fingertip
- Donor site closed primarily

Disadvantages [3, 7, 8]
- It requires a meticulous technique.
- There is a risk of contractures because the flap crosses skin creases.
- Flap failure may cause significant morbidity and a much larger defect than that of the original one, making further reconstruction more complicated.

Marking Technique [2, 3, 5, 6]
- The flap can be designed and raised as either a unilateral or bilateral V-Y advancement neurovascular flap on the lateral aspect (radial or ulnar) of the digit (Fig. 12.1).
- The flap is designed as a triangle:
  - The dorsal limb of the V (the dorsal incision) corresponds to the mid-lateral line of the digit.
  - The volar limb of the V (the sloping anterior "volar" incision) terminates at the wound edge at the midline of the digit.
  - The apex of the V is placed at the DIP joint crease.
- Digital Allen's test and examination with a handheld Doppler to ensure patency of the digital arteries are carried out before the procedure.

Surgical Technique [2, 3, 5, 6]
- The surgery is performed under regional or general anesthesia.
- A tourniquet is applied to the arm.

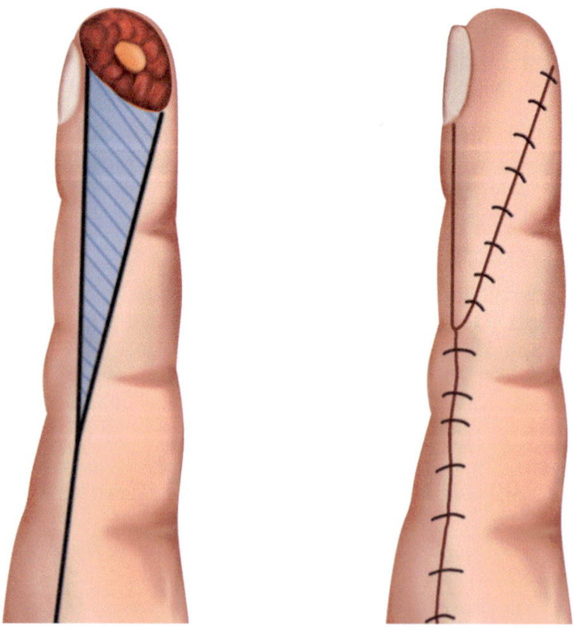

Fig. 12.1 The flap is designed as V-Y along the mid-axial line to include the neurovascular bundle with the apex at the DIP crease. The incision is carried away down to the periosteum while ensuring having the bundle within the flap. Release of the septae and fibrous attachment is done to ease the advancement of the flap

- Debridement of the stump to healthy tissue and removing any contaminated tip of the distal phalanx are conducted.
- After the flap marking is done, an incision is made down to the periosteum in the mid-lateral line (the dorsal incision).
- Dissection is continued medially and proximally from the lateral flap in the plane immediately superficial to the periosteum, with the digital artery being easily followed down the deep surface of the flap.
- The skin overlying the medial limb of the flap is incised (the volar incision) and the subcutaneous tissue is gently spread by dissection scissors.
- Cleland's ligament and the fibrous septa that connect the dermis to the periosteum and tendon sheath are divided to mobilize the flap.
- Care must also be taken not to injure the small venae comitantes and veins present in the subcutaneous tissues surrounding the digital artery and nerve since this might lead to venous congestion.
- The flap is advanced and inset without tension and loosely sutured.
- The donor site is closed primarily. Commonly, part of the mid-lateral margin of the flap is left unsutured to avoid tension.

Postop Care [2, 3, 6, 7]
- A nonadherent dressing is applied.
- The finger is splinted dorsally, with the joint slightly flexed for the first 72 h to take tension off the pedicle. However, this position is not maintained after this time because of the risk of volar plate contracture of the PIP joint.

Complications [2, 3, 6, 7]
- PIP joint flexion contracture
- Cold intolerance in cold climates
- Partial flap necrosis or total flap necrosis
- Hypersensitive scar

Variants
- Lanzetta modification, the flap is extended proximally to the PIP joint crease [2].
- Smith and Elliot modification (extended Segmüller flap), the flap is extended proximally over the middle of the proximal phalanx [3].

References

1. Segmüller G. Modifikation des Kutler-Lappens: neuro-vaskulre stielung. Handchirurgie. 1976;8:75–6.
2. Lanzetta M, Mastropasqua B, Chollet A, Brisebois N. Versatility of the homodigital triangular neurovascular island flap in fingertip reconstruction. J Hand Surg. 1995;20(6):824–9.
3. Smith KL, Elliot D. The extended Segmüller flap. Plast Reconstr Surg. 2000;105(4):1334–46.
4. Tang JB, Elliot D, Adani R, Saint-Cyr M, Stang F. Repair and reconstruction of thumb and finger tip injuries. Clin Plast Surg. 2014;41(3):325–59.

5. Konczalik W, Michno D, Kang N. Locoregional flaps in the hand. Hand Trauma Clin Pract. 2019;8:91–144.
6. Arsalan-Werner A, Brui N, Mehling I, Schlageter M, Sauerbier M. Long-term outcome of fingertip reconstruction with the homodigital neurovascular island flap. Arch Orthop Trauma Surg. 2019;139(8):1171–8.
7. Foucher G, Boulas HJ, Braga Da Silva J. The use of flaps in the treatment of fingertip injuries. World J Surg. 1991;15(4):458–62.
8. Appukuttan A, Ragoowansi R. The unilateral perforator V-Y flap for fingertip reconstruction: a versatile technique. JPRAS Open. 2020;23:1–7.

Part III

Finger-Related Flaps

Standard Cross-Finger (Cronin) Flap 13

Hassan abbas Ali and Turki Alhassan

Classification [1]

- Two-stage flap reconstruction
- Transposition pedicled skin flap

Vascular Supply [1, 2]

- The subdermal vascular plexus located on the dorsum of the digit (deep to the dermis and superficial to the epitenon), originating from the digital arteries
- Flap design as a random pattern
- Flap venous drainage through subcutaneous dorsal veins or the delicate concomitant veins and adventitial veins of the vasa vasorum of the arterial branches

Innervation

- The dorsal skin of the donor site innervated by the dorsal branch of the proper palmar digital nerve (taking off usually at the level of the proximal phalanx base)

Indications [1, 3]

- Any volar soft tissue defect of the fingers (index to small fingers) from the finger pulp to the proximal phalanx
- Palmar oblique defects of the finger pulp (a sensate variant of the cross-finger flap)

Contraindications [4]

- Stiffness or impaired joint motion (e.g., arthritis and contracture)
- Impaired vascular digital circulation (donor site morbidity including traumatic and Raynaud's syndrome)

H. a. Ali · T. Alhassan (✉)
Plastic Surgery Division, Department of Surgery, Ministry of National Guard - Health Affairs, King Abdullah International Medical Research Center, Riyadh, Saudi Arabia

O. Almeshal et al. (eds.), *Soft Tissue Reconstruction of the Hand: Loco-regional and Distant Flaps Selection and Approach*,
https://doi.org/10.1007/978-981-16-9945-0_13

- Not suitable for middle fingertip injury as neighboring fingers are shorter, requiring the middle finger to be in force flexion to fit the next finger

Advantages [4]
- Simple technique
- Good sensate in the sensitive area
- Minimal functional and cosmetic issues

Disadvantages [4]
- Two-stage procedure
- Immobilization leading to stiffness
- Donor site morbidity (stiffness, neuroma, and epithelial cyst)
- Requiring skin graft to cover the donor site.

Marking Technique [1, 5]
- The flap is rectangular and is based on the mid-lateral line closest to the recipient digit (Fig. 13.1).
- The flap is selected from the dorsal aspect of the middle phalanx at a level close to the area of injury in the other digit.
- No flap from the distal phalanx is selected.
- Usually, the digit radial to the injured finger is used as the donor for the flap (e.g., a cross-finger flap raised from the middle finger used as the donor to the ring finger).
- The cross-finger flap may be pedicled laterally, proximally, or distally.
- The flap is limited between PIP and DIP joints.

Surgical Technique [1, 2, 5, 6]
- The patient is placed in the supine position and the upper limb is supported by arm table.
- Surgery can be performed under local or general anesthesia.
- The flap to be raised is designed to be approximately 25% larger than the defect to be reconstructed.
- The flap is designed with two transverse limbs (not violating the IP joints) and one longitudinal limb (at the mid-lateral line away from the recipient digit).
- Recipient finger is debrided.
- Incisions are made through the epidermis and dermis until dorsal veins are seen.
- The superficial skin veins are ligated.
- The defect is widened on both sides.
- Laterally, the skin flap should not exceed the mediolateral line.
- Release of Cleland's ligaments at the base of the flap (undermining flap) will give extra mobility and prevent stretching of the flap.
- Flap dissection is carried out until the connective-tissue layer above the peritendinous tissue of the extensor aponeurosis up to the mediolateral line.
- The skin pedicle is then flipped 180 degrees and transposition is made to cover the skin defect.

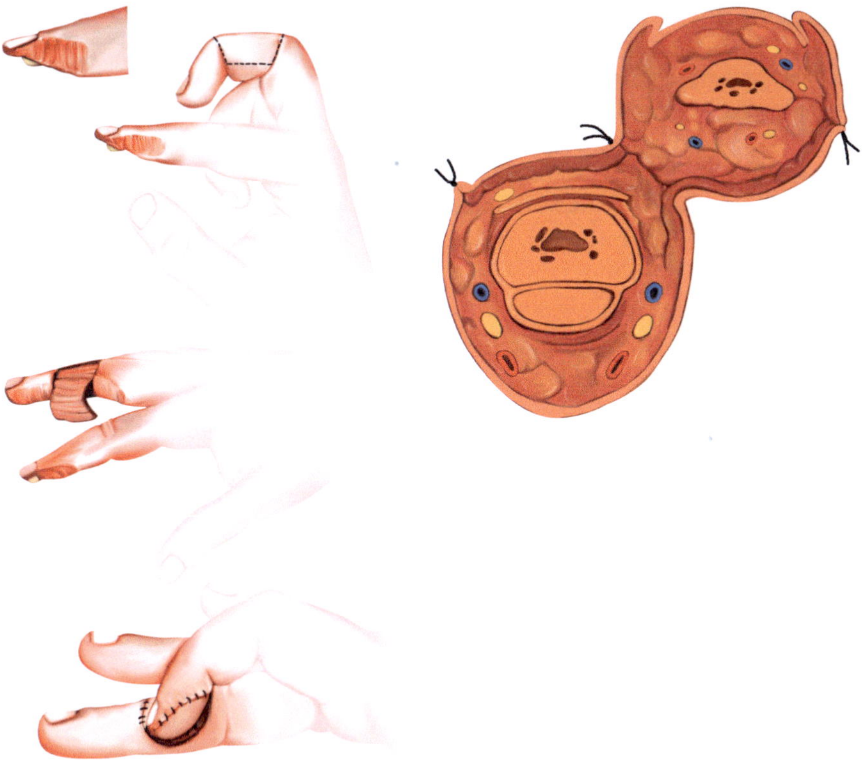

Fig. 13.1 The flap design. The flap is designed over the dorsal aspect of the middle phalanx near to the area of injury in the adjacent digit. The flap location is estimated by flexing the injured digit to approximate the middle phalanx of the donor digit. After the flap is designed, the flap is raised from the dorsum of the digit with dissection over the extensor paratenon with its base ipsilateral to the digit to be covered. The skin flap is then turned over 180 degrees and transposed to cover the defect. The donor site is then skin-grafted. The two fingers are further secured to each other with sutures to prevent flap avulsion

- Then, the tourniquet is released, blood supply is checked, and hemostasis is secured.
- Before the cross-finger flap insetting, a full-thickness skin graft (FTSG) is harvested and sutured over the donor site (the skin graft is first sutured to the lateral margin of the recipient wound to ensure that the subdermal plexus of the cross-finger flap does not sustain an iatrogenic injury while suturing the FTSG).
- The flap is sutured without any tension.
- A tie-over bolster is applied only to the FTSG with a petroleum-based nonadherent dressing.
- K-wire can be inserted across the donor and recipient digits proximal to the injury zone (be careful not to damage the blood supply).
- A plaster splint may also be applied.

- Traditionally, the division of the flap is performed 10–14 days after the first operation, but viability should be tested;
  - After exsanguinating the donor finger with manual pressure, a small Penrose drain is used as a tourniquet at the base of this finger, proximal to the donor flap site. With the tourniquet in place, the flap itself is carefully examined. If the flap has been successfully vascularized by the recipient finger, the capillary refill in the flap will be detectable. Then, the division of the pedicle can be safely performed.

Postop Care [1, 2, 4, 5]
- Flap first dressing at day 7 to assess the flap
- Flap separation at days 14–21
- Flap separation daily dressing of wound to heal by secondary intention

Complications
- Minimal joint stiffness
- Cold intolerance
- Flexion/extension contracture
- Color mismatch
- Asymmetry of reconstructed pulp volume compared to the contralateral finger
- Reconstructed finger variation of static discrimination and tactile discrimination compared to the contralateral finger (sensitivity reappearing at 12–18 months postoperatively)

Variants [2, 6–10]
- Cross-finger flap to cover all four fingers simultaneously (multiple cross-finger flaps, "piggyback" technique)
- Modification of elevation of the cross-finger flap in a plane superficial to the dorsal veins of the fingers (preventing donor site morbidities, such as adhesion, contracture, and contour deformity)
- Microsurgical sensate cross-finger flap according to Berger and Meissl
- Deepithelialized reverse cross-finger flap according to Pakiam
- Modification by using a thin flap of full-thickness skin only
- The cross-finger skin flap to volar finger tissue defect (preserving cutaneous vein and donor site morbidity)

Case

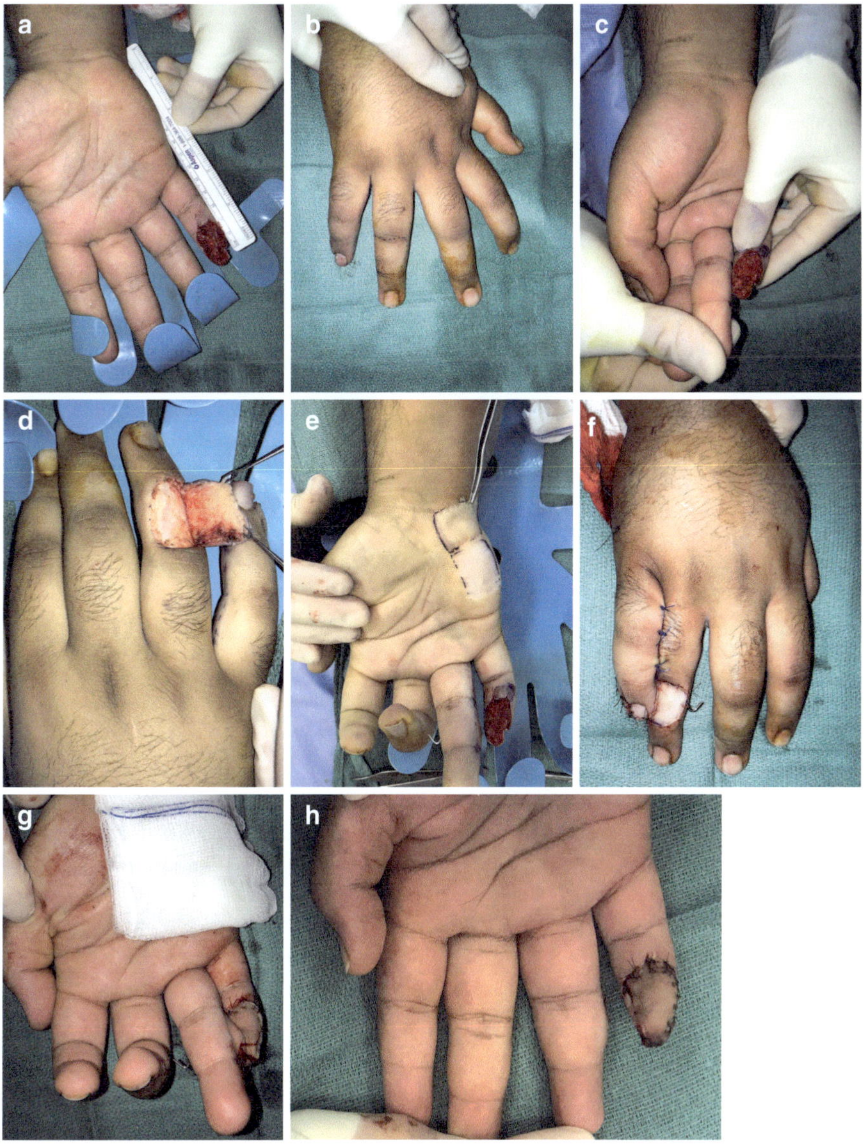

Case 13.1 Intraoperative photos of a patient who presented with soft tissue loss over the volar side of the distal phalanx of little with exposed bone finger as in (**a**). Coverage was planned with cross-finger flap as marked in (**b**, **c**) on the dorsum of the middle phalanx on the ring finger with its base on the ipsilateral side of the defect, making sure it has good reach and alignment with the defect. The flap was then raised, leaving the extensor ton paratenon intact, as seen in (**d**). The flap was then inset to the defect together with securing sutures of the fingers together to protect the flap from avulsion and the donor site was skin-grafted as seen in (**e**–**g**). After 3 weeks, the patient was taken back to the operating room in which the flap was then separated as seen in (**h**)

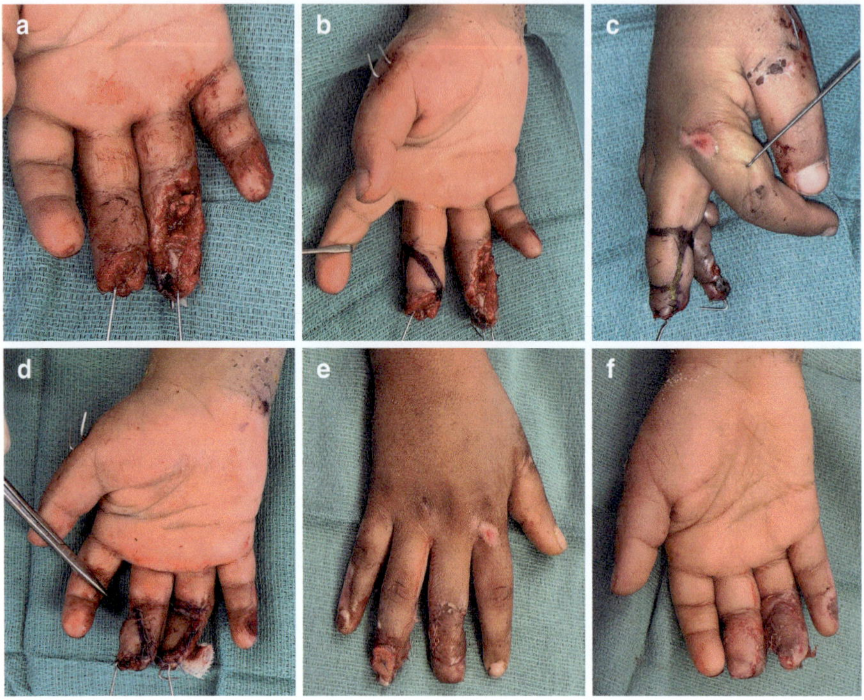

Case 13.2 Intraoperative photos of a patient presented with hand crush injury with soft tissue loss over the middle and ring finger with exposed bone in (**a**). Soft tissue coverage was planned with a combination of cross-finger flap for the coverage of ring finger defect and oblique triangular (Venkataswami) flap for the coverage of middle finger defect, all based on the ring finger as seen in (**b**, **c**), and flaps were then raised and inset to the defect and skin graft was laid over the donor site as in (**d**). Three weeks after that, cross-finger flap was separated with good soft tissue coverage as seen in (**e**, **f**)

References

1. Kappel DA, Burech JG. The cross-finger flap. An established reconstructive procedure. Hand Clin. 1985 Nov;1(4):677–83.
2. Chao JD, Huang JM, Wiedrich TA. Local hand flaps. J Am Soc Surg Hand. 2001 Feb 1;1(1):25–44.
3. Rabarin F, Saint Cast Y, Jeudy J, Fouque PA, Cesari B, Bigorre N, Petit A, Raimbeau G. Cross-finger flap for reconstruction of fingertip amputations: long-term results. Orthop Traumatol Surg Res. 2016 Jun 1;102(4):S225–8.
4. Cronin TD. The cross finger flap: a new method of repair. Am Surg. 1951 May;17(5):419–25.
5. Gudin M, Pangman WJ. The repair of surface defects of fingers by trans-digital flaps. Plast Reconstr Surg. 1950 Apr 1;5(4):368.
6. Ahmed N. Experience of cross finger flap. Esclapio. 2009;5(2)
7. Hastings H. Dual innervated index to thumb cross finger or island flap reconstruction. Microsurgery. 1987;8(3):168–72.

8. Nicolai JP, Hentenaar G. Sensation in cross-finger flaps. Hand. 1981;13(1):12–6.
9. Gokrem S, Tuncali D, Terzioglu A, Toksoy K, Aslan G. The thin cross finger skin flap. J Hand Surg. 2007 Aug;32(4):417–20.
10. Chitta M, Malathi L, Joseph A. Cross-finger flap to the thumb: quest for an alternate donor. Indian J Plast Surg. 2020 Aug;53(2):287–92.

Reverse Cross-Finger Flap 14

Hassan abbas Ali and Turki Alhassan

Classification [1] Regional axial flaps

Vascular Supply [1] Palmar digital arterial network

Innervation [2]
- Anastomosis between the dorsal sensory branch and the pulp branch

Indications [3]
- Dorsal finger soft-tissue defect, from fingertip till the level of the proximal phalanx

Contraindications [3]
- Extensive dorsal skin loss
- Injuries to the adjacent digits

Advantages
- Simple technique
- Good sensibility in the sensitive area
- Minimal functional and cosmetic issues

Disadvantages
- Two-stage procedure
- Immobilization leading to stiffness.
- Donor site morbidity (stiffness, neuroma, and epithelial cyst)
- Requiring recipient site skin grafting

H. a. Ali · T. Alhassan (✉)
Plastic Surgery Division, Department of Surgery, Ministry of National Guard - Health Affairs, King Abdullah International Medical Research Center, Riyadh, Saudi Arabia

O. Almeshal et al. (eds.), *Soft Tissue Reconstruction of the Hand: Loco-regional and Distant Flaps Selection and Approach*,
https://doi.org/10.1007/978-981-16-9945-0_14

Marking Technique [1]

- The flap is obliquely located at the dorsum of the middle phalanx about 1 cm long and about 4–5 mm wider than the defect (Fig. 14.1).
- The longitudinal limb of the flap is marked on the mid-lateral line.
- The mid-lateral line mark will be on the side of the injured digit.

Surgical Technique [1, 3]

- Axillary block or regional anesthesia and arm tourniquet are preferred.
- The thin full-thickness flap is elevated superficial to the subdermal plexus.
- Then, the subcutaneous tissue flap is elevated at the level of the extensor paratenon.
- This elevated subcutaneous flap is now sutured to the defect.
- The originally elevated, thin, full-thickness skin flap is then sutured back to cover the donor defect and a tie-over dressing is applied.
- After good hemostasis is obtained, the reverse surface of the thin subcutaneous flap on the injured finger is covered with a thin FTSG without a tie-over dressing.

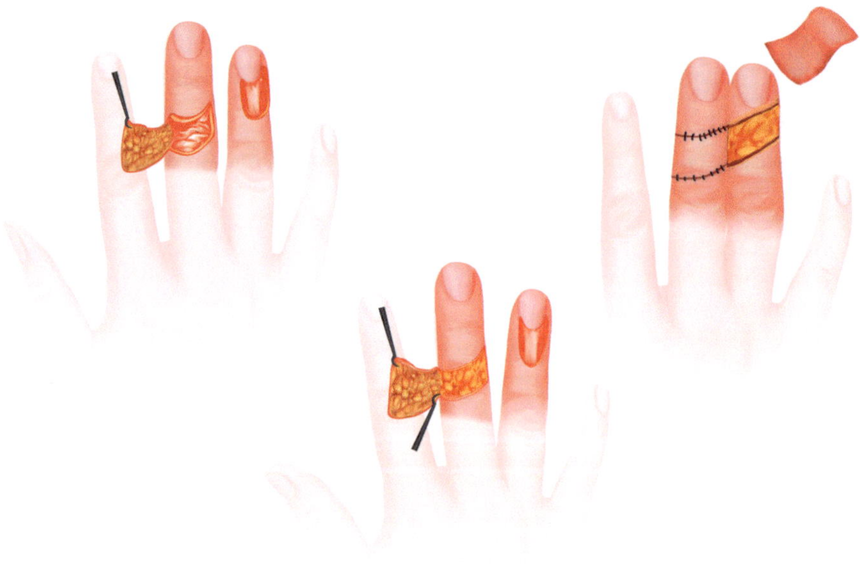

Fig. 14.1 The flap design. The flap is designed over the dorsum of the adjacent finger middle phalanx. A thin skin flap is raised with its base on the contralateral side of the finger to be reconstructed, leaving the subcutaneous tissue intact. Next, a subcutaneous tissue adipofascial flap is raised with its base on the ipsilateral side of the finger to be reconstructed. This flap is then flipped and inset to the dorsal finger defect. After flap insetting, a split-thickness skin graft is then applied over the mobilized flap and the raised thin skin flap of the donor site is applied back. The fingers are then sutured to each other to protect the flap from avulsion

Postop Care [1, 2, 4, 5]

- Extremity elevation in a sling is important.
- Dressing and sutures are removed in about 2 weeks.
- Slight venous congestion at the flap may show in 2 days, requiring leech or release of some sutures.
- Early physiotherapy for the hand is started to prevent stiffness.
- The flap can be divided after 14 days.

Variants [2, 6–11]

- The flap can be used as a sensate pedicle reverse heterodigital cross-finger flap.
- A long pedicle can be dissected to reach the dorsoradial side of a recipient finger from an ulnar donor site.
- Spare-part fillet finger flaps are utilized in a cross-finger fashion to reconstruct adjacent complex digital defects.

Case

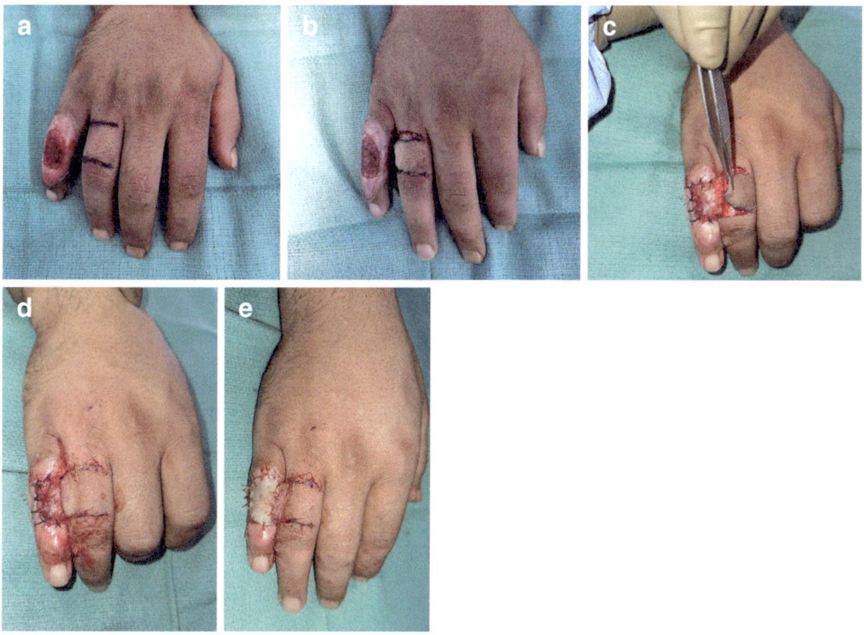

Case 14.1 Intraoperative photo of a patient who presented with a traumatic wound over the dorsum of the middle phalanx and proximal interphalangeal joint of the little finger with soft tissue loss. After ensuring a clean wound, coverage was planned with a reverse cross-finger flap from the dorsum of the adjacent ring finger as marked in (**a**). The procedure started with raising the skin over the flap site with its base attached on the contralateral side of the defect, leaving the dorsal adipofascial tissue intact, as seen in (**b**). After that, the dorsal adipofascial flap was raised over the extensor tendon with its base on the ipsilateral side of the defect and then inset to the defect on the little finger as seen in (**c**). The raised skin flap was then put back and sutured to its place except at the adipofascial flap pedicle attachment side as seen in (**d**). Then, the skin graft was laid over the adipofascial flap, as seen in (**e**)

References

1. Germann G, Rütschle S, Kania N, Raff T. The reverse pedicle heterodigital cross-finger island flap. J Hand Surg. 1997 Feb;22(1):25–9.
2. Lee NH, Pae WS, Roh SG, Oh KJ, Bae CS, Yang KM. Innervated cross-finger pulp flap for reconstruction of the fingertip. Arch Plast Surg. 2012 Nov;39(6):637.
3. Atasoy E. The reverse cross finger flap. J Hand Surg. 2016 Jan 1;41(1):122–8.
4. Alonso-Artieda M. Reimplantation of an avulsed ring finger using a sensory cross-finger flap. Br J Plast Surg. 1971 Jan;1(24):293–5.
5. Nicolai JP, Hentenaar G. Sensation in cross-finger flaps. Hand. 1981 Feb;1:12–6.
6. Gurbuz K, Uzun E, Ozan F. Covering the dorsal finger defect with reverse cross finger flap. J Clin Anal Med. 2016 Mar 1;7(2):262–4.
7. Cohen BE, Cronin ED. An innervated cross-finger flap for fingertip reconstruction. Plast Reconstr Surg. 1983 Nov 1;72(5):688–97.
8. Chao JD, Huang JM, Wiedrich TA. Local hand flaps. J Am Soc Surg Hand. 2001 Feb 1;1(1):25–44.
9. Pakiam AI. The reversed dermis flap. Br J Plast Surg. 1978 Apr 1;31(2):131–5.
10. Al-Qattan MM, Al Mohrij SA. Spare-part fillet cross-finger flaps: a series of two cases. Int J Surg Case Rep. 2019 Jan;1(60):221–3.
11. Atasoy E. Reversed cross-finger subcutaneous flap. J Hand Surg. 1982 Sep 1;7(5):481–3.

15 C-Ring Cross-Finger Flap (Turkist Flap)

Hassan abbas Ali and Turki Alhassan

Classification [1, 2]

- Fasciocutaneous flap
- Random pattern regional flap

Vascular Supply [1, 3]

- Axial pattern cross-finger flap based on one digital vascular bundle either distally or proximally
- The C-ring cross-finger flap drained via digital venae comitantes

Innervation N/A.

Indications [1]

- To cover relatively large defects of the volar and dorsal skin of the fingers
- To cover degloved finger stumps

Contraindications [1]

- An abnormal digital Allen's test

Advantages [1]

- Compared with a standard cross-finger flap, it has a multidirectional and wider rotation arc.
- Its available size is nearly twice as large as a standard cross-finger flap.
- It allows stump coverage without shortening the length of the finger, even in cases with degloved amputation stumps.
- It has an excellent blood supply.

H. a. Ali · T. Alhassan (✉)
Plastic Surgery Division, Department of Surgery, Ministry of National Guard - Health Affairs, King Abdullah International Medical Research Center, Riyadh, Saudi Arabia

O. Almeshal et al. (eds.), *Soft Tissue Reconstruction of the Hand: Loco-regional and Distant Flaps Selection and Approach*,
https://doi.org/10.1007/978-981-16-9945-0_15

Disadvantages [1]

- Two-stage procedure
- Leaving a noticeable scar on the donor finger

Marking Technique [1–3]

- Before the beginning of marking, the vascularity of the donor finger should be insured.
- The donor digit must have two patent digital arteries confirmed by a digital Allen's test or Doppler examination before surgery.
- *Flap selection:*
  - The flap is based on one of the digital vascular bundles and can be based distally or proximally (Fig. 15.1).
  - It is possible to elevate the C-ring flap either distally or proximally on one digital vascular bundle.
  - The digital nerve is not included in the flap.
  - Although the flap is based on the dorsum of the finger, it can include volar skin of the area of the middle phalanx.
  - For a degloving injury, the flap can be sewn to itself to create a cap over the degloved segment defect.

Surgical Technique [1, 2]

- It can be done under general anesthesia or regional anesthesia with the use of a tourniquet without exsanguination.
- The flap is designed around the dorsal and volar surfaces of the middle phalanx as an open ring.
- As with many of these flaps, the dissection plane is just superficial to the paratenon, with care taken to leave the paratenon intact.
- Following the skin incisions, the digital artery and venae comitantes are ligated proximally or distally depending on the pedicle direction of the flap.
- Flap is now raised in the plane deep to subcutaneous fat, keeping the digital artery and venae comitantes with the flap.
- The digital nerve is preserved, while the digital artery and venae comitantes are included in the flap.
- The skin is usually kept over the digital bundle intact to protect the vascular pedicle.
- The whole dorsal surface must be limited to half the width of the finger on the volar aspect.
- It is very important to reserve the skin of the contralateral side and half the volar width of the donor finger to preserve venous and lymphatic drainage of the distal part of the finger.
- Small skin bridge is left intact to protect the digital artery.
- The flap can be made into an island flap to allow for more flap mobility.
- After complete elevation of the flap, the tourniquet is released, the circulation is checked, and hemostasis is obtained.
- The flap is then inset into the recipient defect.

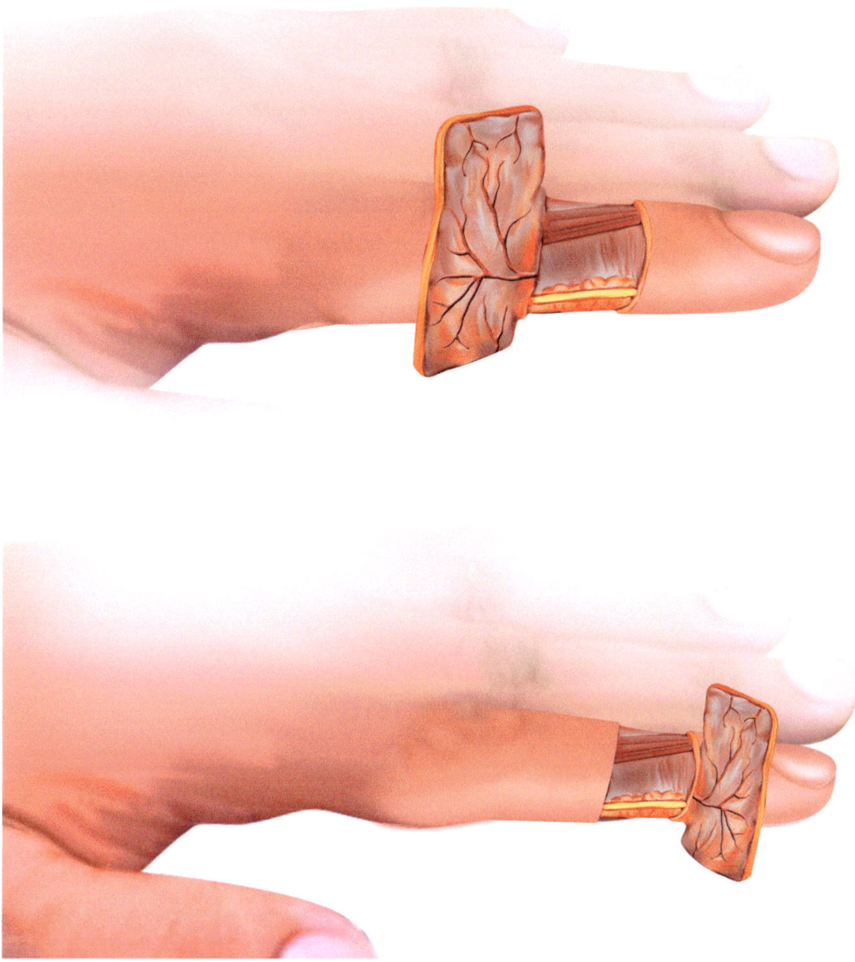

Fig. 15.1 The flap design. The flap is designed on the dorsum of the finger; it can include the volar skin of the area of the middle phalanx. The flap pedicle is based on the digital vascular bundle and can be based distally or proximally. The nerve is not included in the flap elevation. The flap is dissected just superficially to the paratenon. A small skin bridge is left intact to protect the digital artery. The flap is then mobilized to the adjacent finger defect for soft tissue coverage and the donor site is skin-grafted

- A skin graft is used to cover the donor site.
- Light plaster split securely immobilizes the involved fingers, so no aggressive procedure such as K-wire fixation is necessary.

Postop Care [1, 2]
- Flap division is carried out at 10–14 days.
- Then, a light dressing is applied to each finger and active mobilization of the involved and donor fingers is immediately started.
- Physical therapy and scar management are then initiated after complete flap healing.

Complications

- Nerve injury
- Scars
- Flap necrosis

Variants [3]

- Flap design, which lies semi-circumferentially and perpendicular to the vascular axis, usually requires more acute flexion of the finger than does the classical cross-finger technique.
- Island flap is raised from the ulnar aspect of the middle or ring finger based on the ulnar digital neurovascular bundle in order to reconstruct soft tissue defects to the thumb pulp.

References

1. Mutaf M. A new design of the cross-finger flap: the C-ring flap. Br J Plast Surg. 1993 Jan 1;46(2):97–104.
2. Adani R. Heterodigital flaps for severe pulp defects. BMC Proc. 2015 Dec;9(3):1–2.
3. Chao JD, Huang JM, Wiedrich TA. Local hand flaps. J Am Soc Surg Hand. 2001 Feb 1;1(1):25–44.

Dorsal Middle Phalangeal Finger Flap (DMFF)

16

Ahmed T. Al Turki and Turki Alhassan

Classification Fasciocutaneous flap

Vascular Supply [1–5] Dorsal branch of the digital artery and its vena comitans or one of the proper digital arteries (the average diameter of dorsal branch = 0.44 mm).

Innervation Dorsal sensory branch of the proper digital nerve

Indications [1–4]
- Fingertip reconstruction, dorsolateral defect on the adjacent finger, or ipsilateral defect adjacent defects
- Any defect in homodigit or heterodigit that cannot be covered by advancement flap

Contraindications
- Compromised vascular supply
- Extensive dorsal degloving injury
- Smokers

Advantages
- Minimal donor site morbidity
- Single-stage procedure
- Used to fill the cavity and dead space
- Innervated flap

A. T. Al Turki · T. Alhassan (✉)
Plastic Surgery Division, Department of Surgery, Ministry of National Guard - Health Affairs, King Abdullah International Medical Research Center, Riyadh, Saudi Arabia

O. Almeshal et al. (eds.), *Soft Tissue Reconstruction of the Hand: Loco-regional and Distant Flaps Selection and Approach*,
https://doi.org/10.1007/978-981-16-9945-0_16

Disadvantages

- Thin flap
- Developing depigmentation or hyperpigmentation

Marking Technique [2, 3]

- DMFF can be raised on the index, middle, or ring finger. It is most commonly raised on the middle finger.
- DMFF is marked between the mid-lateral lines horizontally and between the metacarpophalangeal joint and distal interphalangeal joint vertically but not including them (Fig. 16.1).
- For the reconstruction of the fingertip of the thumb, index, or middle finger, the flap is raised on the radial digital artery. On the other hand, for the reconstruction of the fingertip of the ring or little finger, the flap is raised on the ulnar digital artery.
- The mid-lateral line is marked (Büchler and Frey dorsal middle phalangeal modified flap is raised on the dorsal branch of the digital artery) with a 5-mm extension palmary (flap raised on the proper digital artery).
- The dorsal digital artery may arise from either the proximal digital artery or the dorsal interosseous metacarpal artery. The proper digital artery gives four dorsal branches, two at proximal and two at middle phalanx almost at the phalanx center.
- The size of the flap is 3.5 × 6 cm.

Surgical Technique [2, 3, 5]

- Under tourniquet, a mid-lateral incision is made and dissection toward the center is carried out.
- The flap is elevated at the paratenon level just over the extensor tendon distally to proximally.

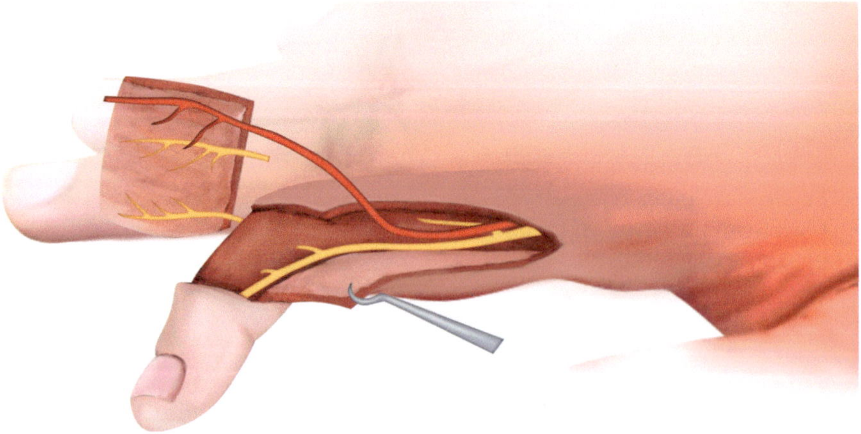

Fig. 16.1 Shows the flap design. The flap is marked on the dorsum of the digit between the mid-lateral lines horizontally. The flap is raised and dissected over the paratenon level. The flap is raised on the dorsal branch of the digital artery and its vena comitans as a pedicle or, if needed, on one of the proper digital arteries. The flap is then transposed to the defect for coverage

- The dorsal sensory nerve is identified and isolated from the neurovascular bundle. Do not isolate the artery in order to preserve the vena comitans.
- In the case of a free flap, the dorsal cutaneous vein is identified and exposed through the central direction.
- The dorsal nerve is cut at the bifurcation site from the digital nerve.
- The distal end of the artery is ligated and cut.
- The flap is now elevated completely with the attached dorsal sensory nerve and proximal pedicel.
- If there is an indication to repair the proper digital artery, a cutaneous vein from the forearm is used as a vein graft to repair the harvested digital artery.
- The tourniquet is released and the flap vascularity is checked.
- A Bruner's zigzag incision is made over the recipient site.
- Vascular supply can be dissected back to the common palmar digital artery or the superficial palmar arch if indicated.
- The distal recipient nerve is refreshed and epineural neurorrhaphy is conducted using 9–0 nylon suture.
- All wounds are closed primarily.
- An FTSG is applied over the donor site. A compression tie-over dressing is applied.
- In the case of a free transfer flap, the digital vein must be isolated and harvested with the flap.

Postop Care

- Light dressing is applied, no pressure over the flap.
- The hand is kept splinted and elevated; active and passive movements are minimized.
- The flap is monitored for congestion, ischemia, and signs of infection.

Complications

- Venous congestion
- Superficial epidermal necrosis that heals well with dressing only
- Hair growth
- Neuroma formation

Variants

- Dorsal branch of digital artery flap
- Proper digital artery flap
- Antegrade flap dissection to a pivot point at the origin of the proper digital artery
- Antegrade flap dissection to a pivot point at the superficial palmar arch
- Harvesting a double DMF flap from two adjacent fingers with the pedicle, including the proper digital artery and their common trunk
- Homodigit application by retrograde dissection to the neck of proximal or middle phalanx or the base of distal phalanx
- Tunneling the flap through intermetacarpal space
- Cross-finger flap
- Free transfer flap

Case

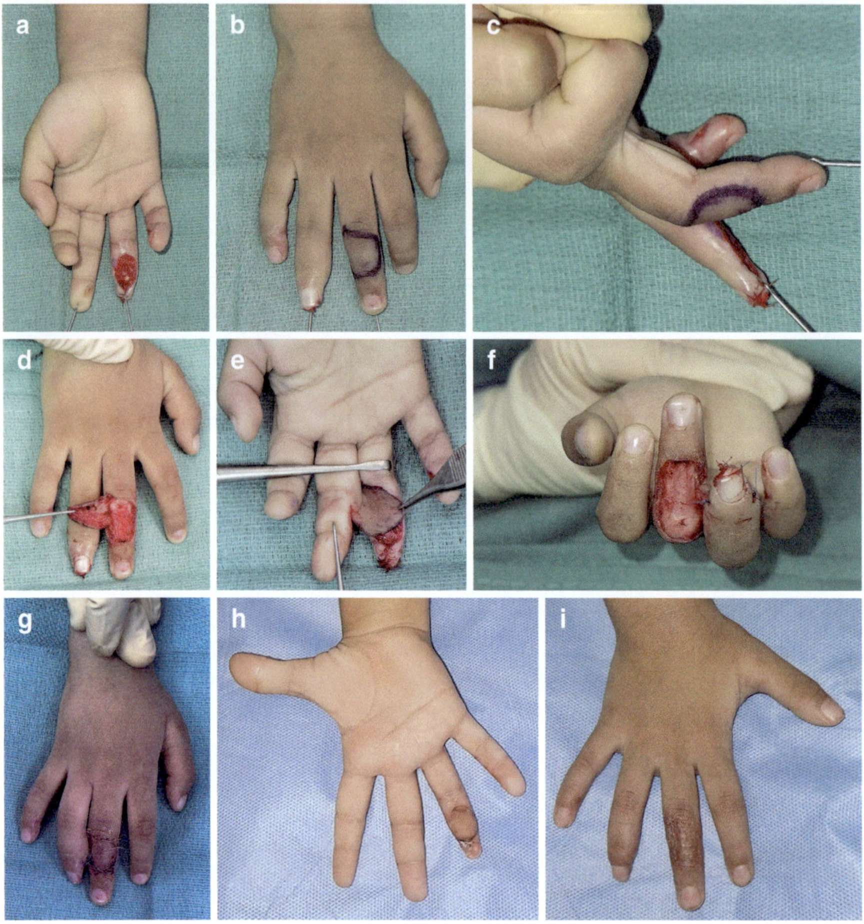

Case 16.1 Intraoperative photo of a patient who presented with ring finger traumatic injury with soft tissue loss over volar distal phalanx and distal interphalangeal joint in (**a**). After good irrigation and washout, coverage was planned with a dorsal middle phalangeal flap from the adjacent ring finger as marked in (**b**, **c**). The flap was then elevated that is based on dorsal branch of the digital artery as seen in (**d**). Flap was then inset and sutured to the defect and donor site was skin grafted as seen in (**e**–**g**). Follow-up assessment at 1 month after flap division is shown in (**h**, **i**) with good soft tissue coverage

References

1. Büchler U, Frey HP. The dorsal middle phalangeal finger flap. Handchir Mikrochir Plast Chir. 1988 Sep 1;20(5):239–43.
2. Hirase Y, Kojima T, Matsuura S. A versatile one-stage neurovascular flap for fingertip reconstruction: the dorsal middle phalangeal finger flap. Plast Reconstr Surg. 1992 Dec;90(6):1009–15.

3. Mahida D. Handbook on flaps in crush injuries of the hand. New Delhi: JP Medical Ltd; 2015.
4. Leupin P, Weil J, Büchler U. The dorsal middle phalangeal finger flap: mid-term results of 43 cases. J Hand Surg Br. 1997 Jun 1;22(3):362–71.
5. Takeishi M, Ishida K, Kurihara K. Free dorsal middle phalangeal finger flap. J Reconstr Microsurg. 2006 Oct;22(07):493–8.

Intercomissural Flap

17

Ahmed T. Al Turki and Turki Alhassan

Classification [1] Fasciocutaneous flap

Vascular Supply [1]

- The dorsal digital artery is a continuation of the dorsal metacarpal artery.
- Palmar digital artery gives off branches communicating with dorsal digital artery: first branch at the level of the middle proximal phalanx; the second branch at the distal third of the proximal phalanx; the third branch at the middle of the middle phalanx; the fourth branch at the level of the distal interphalangeal joint. The diameter of these branches ranges from 0.2 to 0.6 mm.

Innervation Non-innervated flap

Indications

- Coverage of dorsal middle or distal phalanx defect
- Coverage of palmar proximal or middle phalanx defect

Contraindications [2]

- Injury associated with comminuted fractures of the phalanges
- Compromised vascular supply
- Degloving injuries
- Smokers

Advantages [2]

- Minimal donor site morbidity
- Single-stage procedures

A. T. Al Turki · T. Alhassan (✉)
Plastic Surgery Division, Department of Surgery, Ministry of National Guard - Health Affairs, King Abdullah International Medical Research Center, Riyadh, Saudi Arabia

O. Almeshal et al. (eds.), *Soft Tissue Reconstruction of the Hand: Loco-regional and Distant Flaps Selection and Approach*,
https://doi.org/10.1007/978-981-16-9945-0_17

- Pliable, can be turned in any direction; used to fill the cavity and dead space
- Developing sensation

Disadvantages [2]
- Thin flap
- Developing depigmentation or hyperpigmentation
- Developing stiffness if applied over the joint

Marking Technique [2, 3]
- The size of the defect is measured.
- The estimated sites of communication branches of the palmar and dorsal digital artery are marked dorsally. Any site can be used as a pivot point based on the defect site (Fig. 17.1).

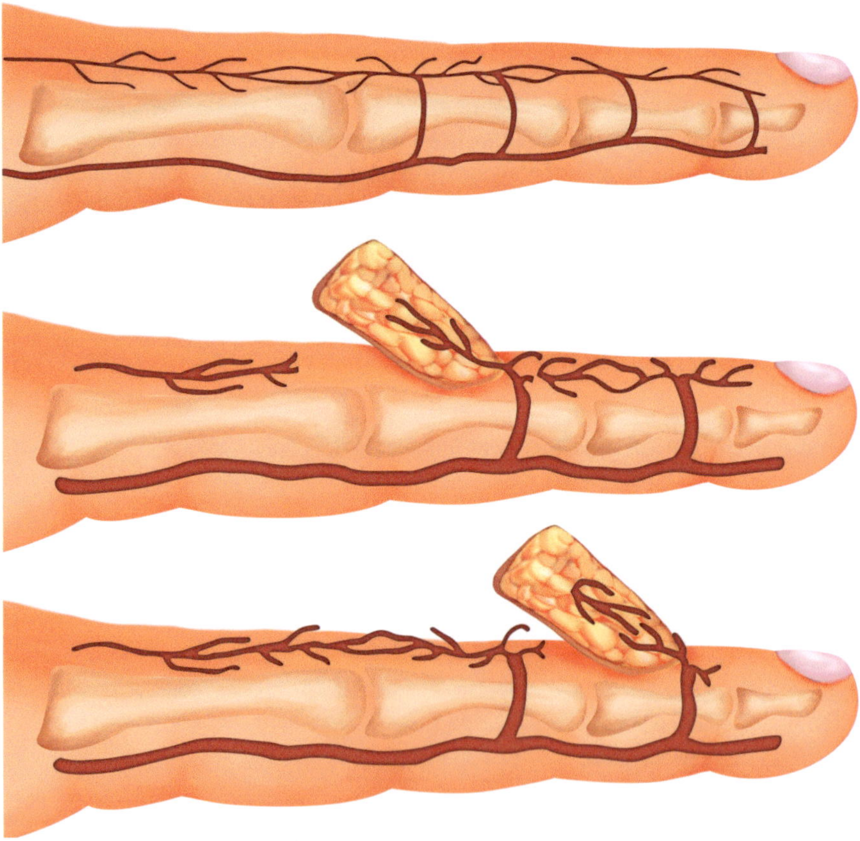

Fig. 17.1 The different locations of the communicating branches of the palmar and dorsal digital artery. Various vessel locations include the following: at the level of the middle proximal phalanx; at the distal third of proximal phalanx; at the middle of the middle phalanx; at the level of the distal interphalangeal joint. The proposed flap is then marked over the dorsum of the finger with the base of the flap at the chosen communicating branch location. The flap is elevated at the paratenon level just over the extensor tendon with a cuff of subcutaneous tissue that protects the flap pedicle

- The subcutaneous pedicle should be as wide as the skin paddle for safety.
- An "S" incision mark is made from the defect that runs proximally to the donor site over the metacarpal or phalanx.

Surgical Technique [2, 3]

- Under tourniquet and local anesthesia, a lazy "S" incision over the pedicle is made through the dermis from the defect to the donor site.
- The skin is undermined and retracted laterally.
- The flap is elevated at the paratenon level just over the extensor tendon as bulk with preservation of subcutaneous tissue. Medial and lateral edges are as long as the flap pedicle.
- It is elevated proximally to distally until reaching the pivot point.
- Avoid visualizing the pedicle not to harm the vessels.
- The tourniquet is released while the flap is in a natural position and the vascularity is visualized.
- The flap is rotated into the defect and fixed with a few stitches.
- Donor site is closed primarily with a skin graft.

Postop Care

- On day 5 or later, whether other injuries exist, a compression dressing is used to prevent venous congestion and bulking of the flap.
- After 2 weeks, active ROM is allowed if not associated with tendon repair.

Complications

Venous congestion

Variants

- Dorsal middle phalangeal flap
- Rotation flap

Case

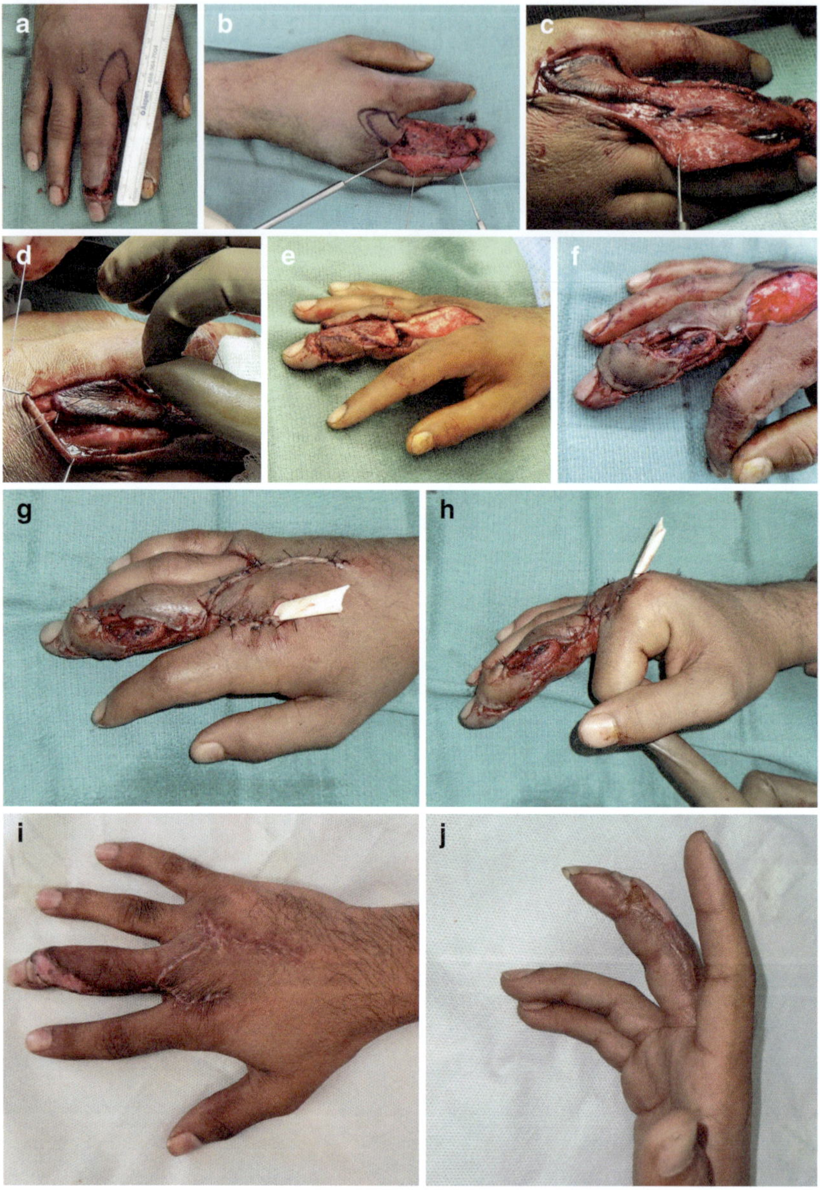

Case 17.1 Intraoperative photo of a patient who presented with middle finger soft tissue loss after a history of snake bite-related finger compartment after decompression. Clean wound coverage was planned with intercommissural flap as marked in (**a**). The procedure started with elevating the skin over the dorsum of the finger, leaving the adipofascial tissue intact, as seen in (**b**). The flap was then elevated proximally to distally with an adipofascial pedicle that contained the dorsal digital artery as seen in (**c**) and the continuation of the dorsal metacarpal artery as ligated as seen in (**d**). The flap was then rotated and inset to the defect as seen in (**e**, **f**). The donor site was closed with a random transposition flap as seen in (**g**, **h**). Follow-up assessment at 2 months after the procedure is seen in (**i**, **j**) with good healing and intact soft tissue coverage

References

1. Valenti P, Masquelet AC, Begue T. Anatomic basis of a dorsocommisural flap from the 2nd, 3rd, and 4th intermetacarpal spaces. Surg Radiol Anat. 1990;12:23.
2. Keramidas E, Rodopoulou S, Metaxotos N, Panagiotou P, Iconomou T, Ioannovich J. Reverse dorsal digital and intercommissural flaps used for digital reconstruction. Br J Plast Surg. 2004 Jan 1;57(1):61–5.
3. Pelissier P, Casoli V, Bakhach J, Martin D, Baudet J. Reverse dorsal digital and metacarpal flaps: a review of 27 cases. Plast Reconstr Surg. 1999;103:159.

18 Homodigital Bipedicled Island Advancement (O'Brien) Flap

Ahmed T. Al Turki and Turki Alhassan

Classification [1–3] Fasciocutaneous bipedicled advancement flap

Vascular Supply Bilateral digital arteries

Innervation Bilateral digital nerves

Indications [1–3]
- Fingertip reconstruction, finger pulp injury, middle volar phalanx reconstruction, restoration of fingertip sensation, and after digital tip neuroma excision

Contraindications
- Compromising palmar vascularity
- Extensive palmar degloving injury
- Smoking

Advantages
- Covering large defects
- Sensate flap
- Reliable blood supply
- Minor donor defect
- No joint contracture
- No danger of dorsal blood supply
- Bipedicle
- Single-stage procedure

A. T. Al Turki · T. Alhassan (✉)
Plastic Surgery Division, Department of Surgery, Ministry of National Guard - Health Affairs, King Abdullah International Medical Research Center, Riyadh, Saudi Arabia

O. Almeshal et al. (eds.), *Soft Tissue Reconstruction of the Hand: Loco-regional and Distant Flaps Selection and Approach*,
https://doi.org/10.1007/978-981-16-9945-0_18

Disadvantages

- Donor site requires skin graft.
- Movement is unidirectional.
- If ischemia occurs, bilateral blood supply is lost.

Marking Technique [1–3]

- The bilateral mid-lateral line is marked from the tip of the finger to the proximal interphalangeal joint crease. If more advancement is needed, the proximal metacarpophalangeal joint crease can be marked (Fig. 18.1).
- The flap can be advanced 1.5 cm distally.

Surgical Technique [1–3]

- The recipient's fingertip is prepped.
- Under tourniquet, the bilateral mid-lateral line is incised.
- The flap is elevated just above the flexor sheath without injury to the flexor sheath.
- The radial and ulnar neurovascular bundles are isolated.
- A transverse incision is made at the desired level while preserving the bilateral neurovascular bundle and then advancing the flap distally. The bundles can be separated from the volar skin by a cannula introduced transversally to easily separate the neurovascular bundle. The cannula is then turned 180 degrees toward the hollow side. Then, the palmer skin can be cut safely [4].

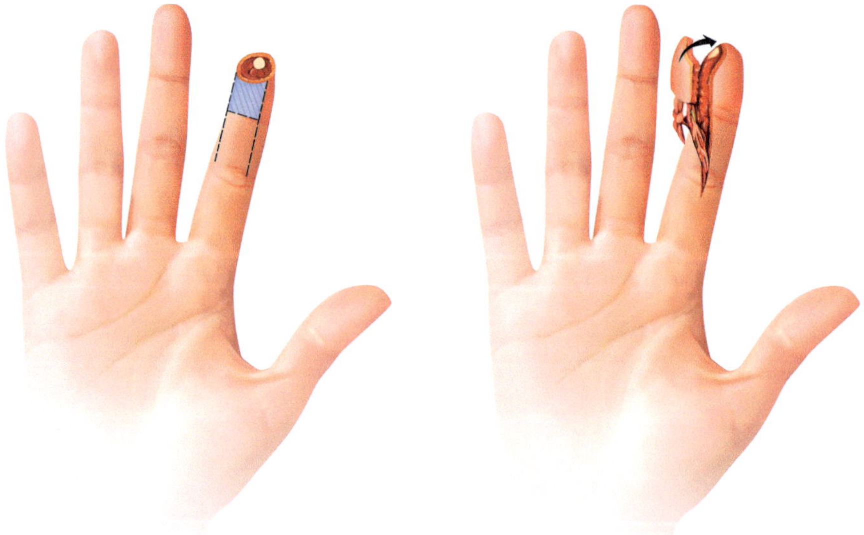

Fig. 18.1 The proposed flap marking. Two bilateral mid-lateral lines are marked starting from the fingertip till the proximal interphalangeal crease. The flap is then elevated just above the flexor sheath. During flap elevation, the radial and ulnar neurovascular bundles are isolated. The flap is then advanced distally while preserving the bilateral neurovascular bundle and then inset to the defect at the fingertip

- The flap is attached distally and sutured.
- If the proximal wound cannot close primarily, a FTSG is used.
- The tourniquet is released and the vascularity is assessed.
- The dressing is applied and a splint is used in mild flexion of the distal and proximal interphalangeal joint for 10 days.

Postop Care
- A light dressing is applied, with no pressure over the flap.
- The hand is kept splinted and elevated; active and passive movements are minimized.
- The flap is monitored for congestion, ischemia, and signs of infection.

Complications [1]
- The full round shape of the pulp beyond the nail margin cannot be achieved due to flat pulp, which does not compromise function.
- Damages to either digital vessel, contracture, or fingertip necrosis are considered contraindications for the flap.

Variant
V-Y advancement flap

References

1. O'Brien B. Neurovascular pedicle transfers in the hand. Aust N Z J Surg. 1965 Aug;35(1):1–1.
2. O'Brien B. Neurovascular island pedicle flaps for terminal amputations and digital scars. Br J Plast Surg. 1968 Jan 1;21(2–3):258–61.
3. Chao JD, Huang JM, Wiedrich TA. Local hand flaps. J Am Soc Surg Hand. 2001 Feb 1;1(1):25–44.
4. Choughri H, Sommier B, Pelissier P. A technical tip of the O'Brien volar advancement flap for thumb reconstruction. J Plast Reconstr Aesthet Surg. 2009 Jun;62(6):e176–7. https://doi.org/10.1016/j.bjps.2008.09.022.

Homodigital Quadrangular Flap (Heuston Flap)

19

Ezekwe E. Amirize and Turki Alhassan

Classification [1] Rotation advancement flap (a lateral palmar advancement flap)

Vascular Supply [1–3]

- An arterial flap originates from the digital artery, perfused by its cutaneous perforators.
- Digital artery derives from a neurovascular bundle included at the flap base; it could be either radial or ulnar.
- Venous drainage is via subdermal venous plexus and venae comitantes.

Innervation [2] A proper digital nerve

Indications [2, 4–7]

- Amputation of the tip of hand digits where replantation is not possible and coverage with a sensate tissue is desired.
- Fingers and thumb palmer pulp tissue loss when bone length preservation and avoidance of nail deformity are necessary.
- Suitable for type 1 (guillotine/transverse) and type 2 oblique amputations.

Contraindications [2, 6]

- Neurovascular bundles injury in the digit.
- Loss of palmer homodigital tissue, for example, crush injury.
- When more than 1.8 cm of tissue advancement is required.

E. E. Amirize · T. Alhassan (✉)
Plastic Surgery Division, Department of Surgery, Ministry of National Guard - Health Affairs, King Abdullah International Medical Research Center, Riyadh, Saudi Arabia

O. Almeshal et al. (eds.), *Soft Tissue Reconstruction of the Hand: Loco-regional and Distant Flaps Selection and Approach*,
https://doi.org/10.1007/978-981-16-9945-0_19

Advantages [2–7]

- Providing glabrous tissue cover for fingertip defect.
- One-stage procedure, with simple and quick dissection.
- Modifiable to close flap volar defect and to increase advancement.
- Bone length preservation.
- Less risk of skin slough on the dorsum of the finger as only one neurovascular bundle is raised with the flap.

Disadvantages [2–7]

- It is unable to achieve more than 2 cm flap advancement.
- It is liable to produce parrot beak nail deformity due to traction.
- The technique can be complicated with scar entrapment and painful neuromas.
- Cold intolerance of digit may occur and tends to persist.
- Flap advancing edge, which is devoid of a digital nerve, is insensate immediately after reconstruction. Hence, a mid-axial incision should be placed on the non-dominant pulp to preserve sensation on the dominant pulp.
- Sensory recovery on the advanced flap edge without a neurovascular bundle is slow and incomplete. However, this can be deployed to treat painful neuroma in an amputation stump by mid-axial incision placement on the neuroma side to provide an insensate skin cover of the neuroma.

Marking Technique [5–7]

- An L-shaped marking is done for an L-shaped incision.
- The longitudinal limb of the "L" is marked on the mid-lateral line of the digit from the fingertip defect to the proximal interphalangeal (PIP) joint flexion crease. This limb is marked on the nondominant (less functional) side of the finger or thumb (Fig. 19.1).
- The transverse limb is marked across the PIP joint flexion crease.
- In a variant, a triangular rotation flap is marked proximally along the mid-lateral incision for closure of the volar flap donor defect.
- The longitudinal limb can also be extended to the metacarpophalangeal (MCP) joint flexion crease.

Surgical Technique [1, 2, 5, 7–9]

- With the patient lying supine with hand on arm table, under local, regional, or general anesthesia, marking is made.
- Debridement of finger or thumb tip injury is done.
- The procedure is done under loupe magnification.
- According to marking, incisions are made.
- A longitudinal incision is made from the defect to the appropriate flexion crease.
- A transverse incision is made on the flexion crease across the finger.
- Flap dissection is done superficially to the neurovascular bundle distally to proximally along the mid-lateral incision.
- Dissection then proceeds above the flexor tendon sheath to the contralateral neurovascular bundle included in the flap by dissecting deep into it.

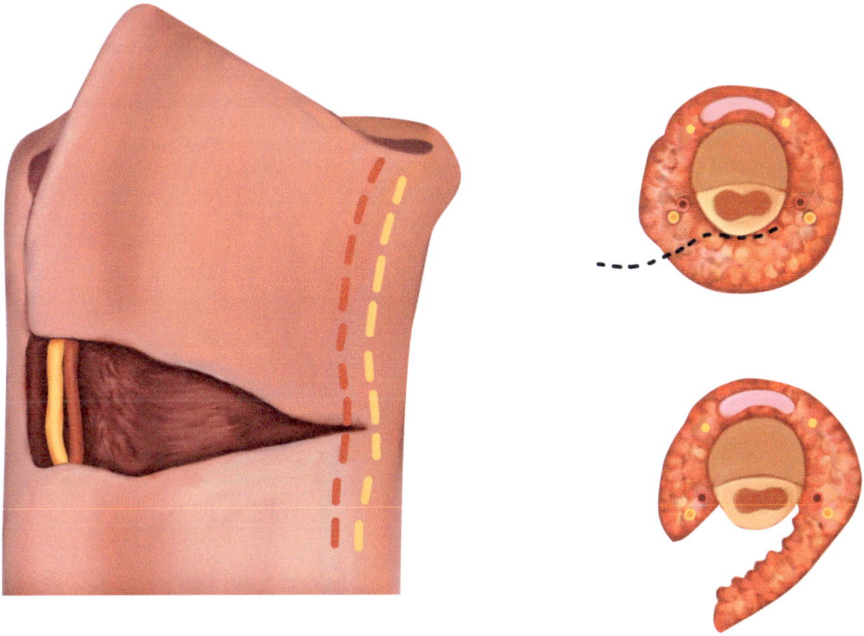

Fig. 19.1 The proposed flap design. An L-shaped line is marked over the mid-axial line of the digit. A transverse limb is then marked across the PIP joint flexion crease. The flap is then dissected superficially to the neurovascular bundle. This is done in a distal to proximal fashion along the mid-lateral incision. Next, the dissection is carried above the flexor tendon sheath to the contralateral neurovascular bundle included in the flap by going deep into it. The flap is then rotated to the distal defect and the donor site is skin grafted

- When elevated completely, the flap is then advanced and rotated to the pulp defect.
- The neurovascular bundle included in the flap can be dissected further proximally to release tension for more flap advancement.
- Flap donor defect can be allowed to heal by secondary intention, closed with a split or a full-thickness skin graft or triangular flap transposition.
- The triangular flap donor site is closed primarily.

Postop Care
- Wound care.
- Evaluation of flap and digit vascularity in the immediate postoperative period.
- Hand immobilization with bulky dressings for 7–10 days.
- Active/passive ROM.

Complications [2, 3, 6]
- Primary or secondary PIP joint contracture.
- Poor sensation in advanced skin.
- Painful neuroma from scar entrapment.
- Dog ear deformity distally.

- Parrot beak nail deformities.
- Diminished flap sensibility when skin graft is placed proximally over the pedicle.
- Cold intolerance.

Variants [2, 6, 8, 10]

- Souquet flap
- Extended Hueston flap:
  - The flap is marked and elevated as originally described, but the flap is extended proximally with a triangular design, radially on the mid-lateral line. This distally based triangular flap is rotated to cover the raw area left after flap advancement.

Case

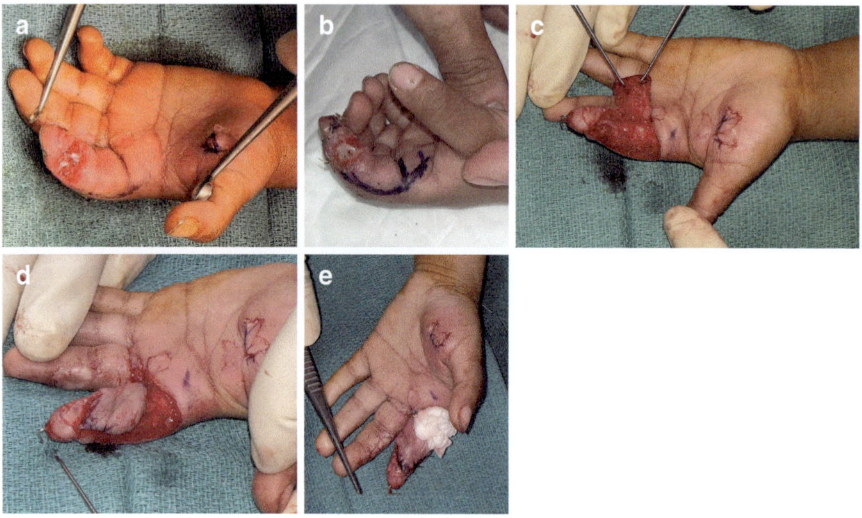

Case 19.1 Intraoperative photo of a patient who presented with index finger volar soft tissue defect with exposed tendons in (**a**). Wound irrigation and washout coverage were planned with a volar homodigital quadrangular flap (Heuston flap) marked in (**b**). The flap was then elevated based on the contralateral cutaneous perforators of the digital artery as seen in (**c**) and then rotated and inset to cover the defect with skin graft applied to cover the donor site as seen in (**d**, **e**)

References

1. Chao JD, Huang JM, Wiedrich TA. Local hand flaps. J Am Soc Surg Hand. February 2001;1(1):25–44.
2. Slutsky DJ. Neurosensory pedicled flaps to the hand. Atlas Hand Clin. 2005;10:141–70.
3. Ganchi PA, Lee PA. Fingertip reconstruction. In: Mathes SJ, editor. Plastic surgery 2nd ed. The hand and upper limb part 1. Philadelphia: Elsevier; 2006. p. 162.
4. Martinez FM, Llanos Guerrero Navarro M, Navarro JG, Ros AG, Robledano AI. Hand coverage. In: Amr S, editor. Issues in flap surgery. London: InTech; 2018.
5. Sokol AB, Berggren RB. Fingertip amputations – review of the procedures and applications. Calif Med. 1973;119:22–8.
6. Foucher G, Boulas HJ, Da Silva JB. The use of flaps in the treatment of fingertip injuries. World J Surg. 1991;15(4):458–62.
7. Dhiren M. Souquet flap. In: Mahida D, editor. Handbook on flaps in crush injuries of the hand. New Delhi: Jaypee Brothers; 2015. p. 40.
8. Brambullo T, Veneza ED, Vindigni V, Bassetto F. Extended Hueston flap: new solution for primary closure. J Hand Microsurg. 2018;10:155–7.
9. Alpar A, Gal A, Patonay L, Kalman M. Local flaps for fingertip injuries: a plastinated model. J Int Soc Plastination. 2001;16:42–5.
10. Lloyd N, Sammut D. A modification of the Souquet advancement flap in fingertip reconstruction. J Hand Surg Eur. 2013 May;38(4):395–8.

Souquet Flap

20

Ezekwe E. Amirize and Turki Alhassan

Classification [1, 2] Rotation advancement flap.

Vascular Supply [1–6]
- Digital artery from both radial and ulnar neurovascular bundles of the digit.
- Venous drainage through their venae comitantes and subdermal venous plexus.

Innervation [1–5]
- Radial and ulnar proper digital nerves.

Indications [3, 6]
- Volar coverage in distal pulp loss.

Contraindications [4]
- Damage to the neurovascular bundle.
- Extensive skin loss (e.g., avulsion).
- Mutilating injuries of the digit.

Advantages [2–6]
- Providing glabrous tissue cover for fingertip defect.
- Modifiable to improve flap advancement.
- Better flap sensitivity (not significantly superior to Hueston flap after long-term follow-up, 3 years and above).
- Helping bone length preservation when advanced.

E. E. Amirize · T. Alhassan (✉)
Plastic Surgery Division, Department of Surgery, Ministry of National Guard - Health Affairs, King Abdullah International Medical Research Center, Riyadh, Saudi Arabia

O. Almeshal et al. (eds.), *Soft Tissue Reconstruction of the Hand: Loco-regional and Distant Flaps Selection and Approach*,
https://doi.org/10.1007/978-981-16-9945-0_20

Disadvantages [1, 3, 4, 6]
- Requiring intact ulnar and radial neurovascular bundles
- Less advancement compared to Hueston flap

Marking Technique [6]
- Like the Hueston flap, an L-shaped incision line is marked with the longitudinal limb on the mid-axial line of the digit, dorsal to the neurovascular bundle (Fig. 20.1).
- The transverse limb is drawn volar across the finger at the proximal interphalangeal joint (PIPJ) crease, extended to the opposite mid-axial line.
- A back cut is marked at this point.

Surgical Technique [1, 3, 4, 6]
- The patient is laid in the supine position with the arm abducted on the table.
- Flap marking is done.
- The procedure is carried out under regional or general anesthesia with loupe magnification.
- The wound bed is prepared by surgical debridement.
- The longitudinal incision is made dorsal to the neurovascular bundle from the defect proximally to the PIPJ flexion crease.
- Next, the transverse incision is made across the flexion crease and extended to the opposite mid-axial line to end in a back cut, with care to preserve the vessels.
- The flap is elevated by dissecting deep to both neurovascular bundles and above the flexor tendon sheath.
- The flap is then advanced to the defect and inset.
- Unlike the Hueston flap, Souquet flap includes the neurovascular bundle in its free edge and thus achieves a lesser advancement.

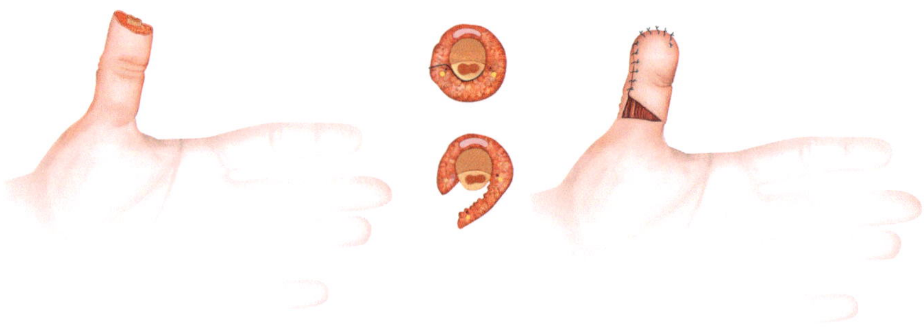

Fig. 20.1 The proposed flap design. An L-shaped incision line is marked with the longitudinal limb on the mid-axial line of the digit, making sure this line is dorsal to the neurovascular bundle. A transverse incision is then made across the flexion crease and is extended to the opposite mid-axial line to end in a back cut, making sure to preserve the vessels. After that, the flap is elevated deep into and including the ipsilateral neurovascular bundle and above the flexor tendon sheath. The raised flap is then rotated distally to cover the fingertip defect and the donor site is skin grafted

Postop Care [5]

- Nonadherent gauze dressing on the flap is applied as the contact layer.
- Fluffed gauze between fingers will prevent maceration.
- Hand is immobilized with bulky dressing in position of function.
- In adults and older children, sutures are removed (e.g., 5/0 nylon) at day 10 postoperatively.
- In younger children, 5/0 Vicryl Rapide or chromic catgut is preferred.
- Physiotherapy/occupational therapy is commenced as necessary.

Variants [3, 6, 7]

- Hueston flap
- N. Lloyd and D. Sammut modification:
  - The Souquet flap is raised in the standard manner: an extension is made of the leading edge incision in the mid-lateral line, enabling dissection, and mobilization of the neurovascular bundle and allowing increased mobility while maintaining full sensibility.
- Marco Roberto Correia Duarte modification:
  - A mid-lateral line is marked from the amputation stump to a point just distal to the metacarpophalangeal joint. The flap was elevated to the palm at the level of the A1 pulley. Along the ulnar border, Grayson's ligaments are identified and dissected to preserve the trifurcation of the distal ulnar digital nerve and to release the vessel that tethers the skin flap proximally. This step increases flap mobility distally and provides a tension-free glabrous cover for the fingertip.

References

1. Chao JD, Huang JM, Wiedrich TA. Local hand flaps. J Am Soc Surg Hand. February 2001;1(1):25–44.
2. Souquet R. The asymmetric arterial advancement flap in distal pulp loss (modified Hueston's flap). Ann Chir Main. 1985;4(3):233–8.
3. Lloyd N, Sammut D. A modification of the Souquet advancement flap in fingertip reconstruction. J Hand Surg Eur. 2013 May;38(4):395–8.
4. Dhiren M. Souquet flap. In: Mahida D, editor. Handbook on flaps in crush injuries of the hand. New Delhi: Jaypee Brothers; 2015. p. 40.
5. Sokol AB, Berggren RB. Fingertip amputations – review of the procedures and applications. Calif Med. 1973 Aug;119:22–8.
6. Slutsky DJ. Neurosensory pedicled flaps to the hand. Atlas Hand Clin. 2005;10:141–70.
7. Correia Duarte MR, Loh CYY, Ahmad Z. The modified Souquet flap for reconstruction of fingertip amputations. Int Wound J. 2018 Aug;15(4):673–4.

Thenar Flap

21

Anas M. Alyamani and Turki Alhassan

Classification [1] Regional fasciocutaneous flap

Vascular supply Random pattern flap

Innervation [1] Neither sensory nor motor nerves are included within the flap, but almost all patients regain functional levels of sensibility, with a mean 2PD of 7 mm.

Indications The thenar flap is indicated for volar skin defect over the pulp of the index or long finger.

Contraindications [2]
- Diseases that increase the risk of developing stiffness, such as arthritis and Dupuytren's contracture.

Advantages [3]
- Hidden donor site defect
- Matching soft tissue thickness and color

A. M. Alyamani · T. Alhassan (✉)
Plastic Surgery Division, Department of Surgery, Ministry of National Guard - Health Affairs, King Abdullah International Medical Research Center, Riyadh, Saudi Arabia

O. Almeshal et al. (eds.), *Soft Tissue Reconstruction of the Hand: Loco-regional and Distant Flaps Selection and Approach*,
https://doi.org/10.1007/978-981-16-9945-0_21

Disadvantages

- Risk of PIP contracture
- Donor site scarring and tenderness

Marking Technique [2, 3]

- The donor site is found by flexing the injured index or middle finger and placing it against the thenar eminence. Draw a circle around the area of contact [2].
- The width of the flap must be 1.5 to two times the width of the defect (Fig. 21.1).
- An H or inverted U-shaped design is drawn. For H-design, the transverse portion of the H is made at the distal edge of the circle.
- However, the flap design can be determined by the defect and by making a template over the thenar skin, the flap can be proximally, distally, or laterally based de- pending on the defect.

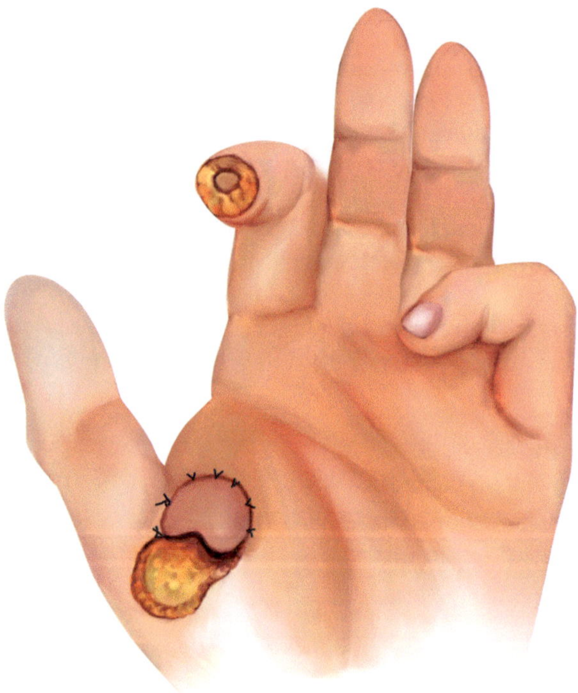

Fig. 21.1 The flap design. In the demonstrated flap, a U-shaped flap design was applied. The flap location was marked by flexing the index finger to the thenar eminence. The flap is then raised in the subcutaneous plane and the donor site is then skin-grafted. The flap is then inset to the defect after flexing the finger toward the flap site

Surgical Technique [2, 3]

- The H- or U-shaped flap design is incised, and the flap is elevated in a subcutaneous plane.
- Care is taken to identify and avoid injury to the radial digital nerve to the thumb. While the thumb is palmary abducted, the finger is fully flexed at the MP joint, and when possible, the distal IP joint is also flexed.
- This results in no more than 40° to 50° of flexion of the proximal IP joint.
- The ends of the flaps are sutured to the respective dorsal and volar fingertips and to each other along the lateral margins.
- This method effectively advances the edges of the donor defects to one another.
- The digit is left attached to the donor site for approximately 2 weeks, and the flap is then divided by using the proximal flap to cover the fingertip and the distal flap to fill in the donor site.
- A skin graft can be applied over the thenar area if it cannot be closed primarily.

Postop Care [3]

- During the first stage, a dorsal block cast is applied to keep the hand immobilized. After the division of the flap's pedicle, active and passive ROM exercises are initiated immediately.

Complications [4]

- Development of proximal interphalangeal joint flexion contractures and persistent tenderness at the flap donor site.

Variants [5, 6]

- Rhomboid or circular flap can be designed based on the shape and size of the finger defect.
- Retrograde neurovascular thenar flap is a sensate variation of thenar flap. It is based on the retrograde flow of the suprafascial branch of the palmar branch of the radial artery. The lateral antebrachial nerve of the forearm is included in the flap and coapted to the digital nerve.

Case

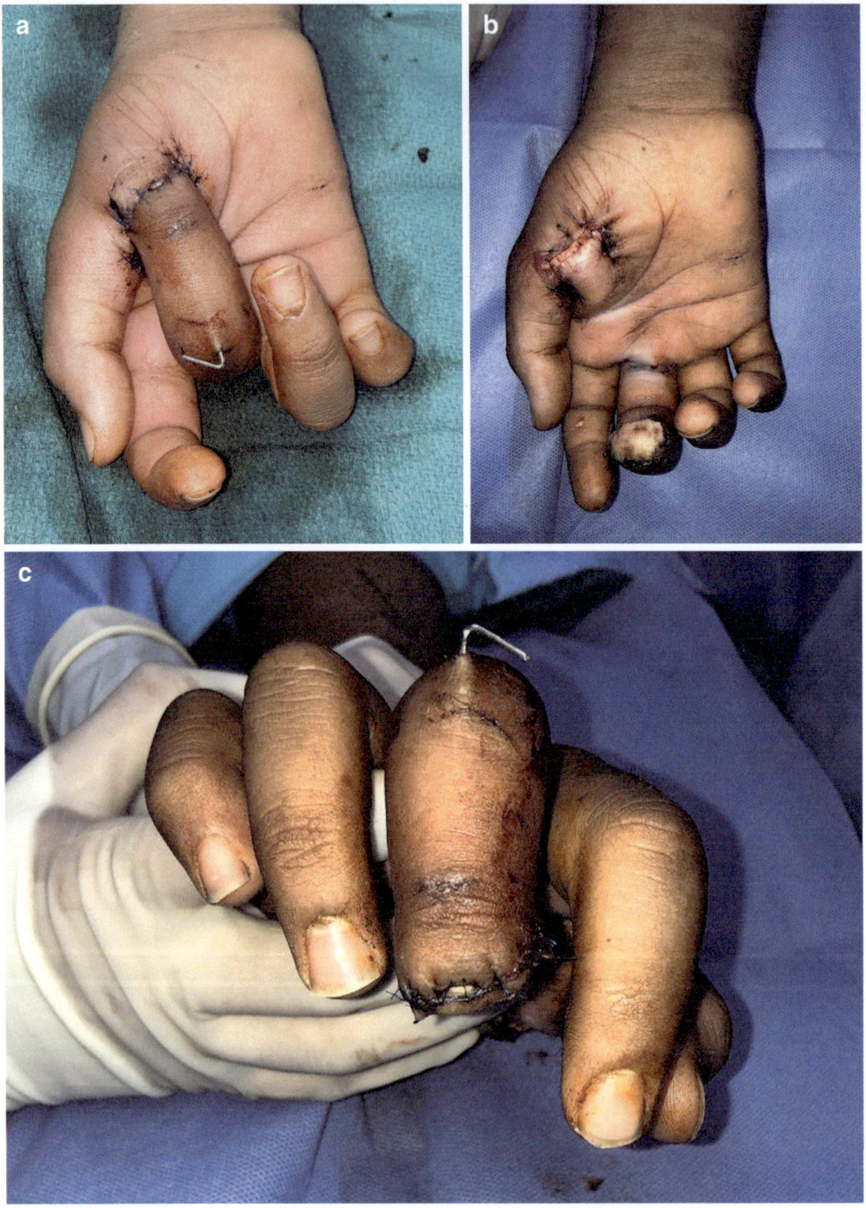

Case 21.1 Intraoperative photo of a patient who presented with middle fingertip injury with exposed bone. The coverage was planned with thenar flap. The flap was designed as a U shape to fit the defect. The finger was then bent and a K-wire was inserted to block the finger in flexion; after that, the flap was inset to cover the defect as seen in (**a**). Three weeks after that, the patient was taken back to the operating room in which the flap was divided after ensuring its good viability and the donor area was primarily closed as seen in (**b**) and (**c**)

References

1. Polatsch DB, et al. The double thenar flap: a technique to reconstruct 2 fingertip amputations simultaneously. J Hand Surg. 2017;42(5):396.e1–5.
2. Chao JD, Huang JM, Wiedrich TA. Local hand flaps. J Am Soc Surg Hand. 2001;1(1):25–44.
3. Melone CP Jr, Beasley RW, Carstens JH Jr. The thenar flap—an analysis of its use in 150 cases. J Hand Surg. 1982;7(3):291–7.
4. Wink JD, et al. Flap reconstruction of the hand. Plastic Reconstruct Surg. 2020;145(1):172e–83e.
5. Rehim SA, Chung KC. Local flaps of the hand. Hand Clinics. 2014;30(2):137–51. v
6. Pediatric thenar flaps: a modified design, case series and review of the literature. J Pediatric Surg. 2013;49(9). https://doi.org/10.1016/j.jpedsurg.2013.11.066

22 Reverse Vascular (Neurovascular) Pedicle Digital Island Flap

Syed M. Ammar Yasir Jaffry

Classification [1–3] Fasciocutaneous flap

Vascular Supply [1–3] Reverse flow in the digital artery is via the middle transverse anastomotic arch between the two digital arteries located at the neck of the middle phalanx in relation to the C3 pulley.

Innervation [1, 4] Sensory innervation is developed through the nerve endings in the bed of the defect. Sensory reinnervation can be attempted utilizing the proper digital nerves or their branches.

Indications [1]
- Defects over the pulp of the finger.
- Dorsal and lateral defects over distal phalanx, DIPJ, middle phalanx, and PIPJ.

Contraindications
- Volar finger defects involving the area of the neck of the middle phalanx.
- Any trauma or defects associated with injury to any of the proper digital vessels (preoperative digital Allen's test can be used to assess the patency of the digital vessels but can be unreliable).

Advantages [2, 4]
- Wide arc of rotation (180 degrees).
- Suitable for large size defects.
- Reliable vascular supply.

S. M. A. Y. Jaffry (✉)
Plastic Surgery Division, Department of Surgery, Ministry of National Guard - Health Affairs, Riyadh, Saudi Arabia

O. Almeshal et al. (eds.), *Soft Tissue Reconstruction of the Hand: Loco-regional and Distant Flaps Selection and Approach*,
https://doi.org/10.1007/978-981-16-9945-0_22

- Minimal donor site morbidity limited to the same digit.
- Single-stage procedure.
- Early mobilization.
- Faster recovery.
- Average sensory recovery (average 2PD of 4–9 mm).

Disadvantages [1, 7]

- The main digital artery sacrificed.
- Flap congestion.
- Donor site skin grafting.
- Flexion contraction at PIPJ level.

Marking Technique [1]

- The patient is placed in a supine position with the arm abducted on the arm table.
- The technique can be done under general anesthesia or regional anesthesia with the use of a tourniquet without exsanguination.
- Digital Allen's test is required to confirm the continuity of the digital vessels and the transverse anastomotic arches, although it can be unreliable.
- The size and shape of the defect are marked and measured and a template is made.
- The flap is marked using the designed template and centered over the digital artery on the dorsolateral aspect of the proximal phalanx (Fig. 22.1).
- The webspace should be avoided in the flap design.
- A small tail can be added to the designed flap distally over the pedicle area to help avoid constriction at the time of flap insetting.
- Zigzag incisions are designed over the longitudinal axis of the pedicle till the defect area.

Surgical Technique [1–3, 5, 6]

- After marking is complete, the tourniquet is inflated, an incision is made through the skin proximally, and the neurovascular bundle is exposed.
- The flap is elevated proximally to distally. Digital nerve is identified and separated from the digital vessels, carefully avoiding injury to the perivascular tissues. Lateral branches of the digital nerve may need to be divided.
- Extreme care is taken while elevating the flap to maintain the continuity of the digital vascular tissue to the overlying skin flap.
- The digital vascular pedicle is dissected from above the flexor tendon sheath and the extensor tendon till 5 mm proximal to DIPJ to avoid injuring the middle transverse communicating arch.
- Skin from the pivot point to the defect area is elevated in the subdermal plane.
- A microvascular clamp is applied to the digital vessels proximal to the proximal part of the flap and the tourniquet is deflated.
- Vascularity to the finger and the flap is observed.
- Once vascularity is confirmed, the vascular clamp is removed and the vascular pedicle is ligated proximally and divided.

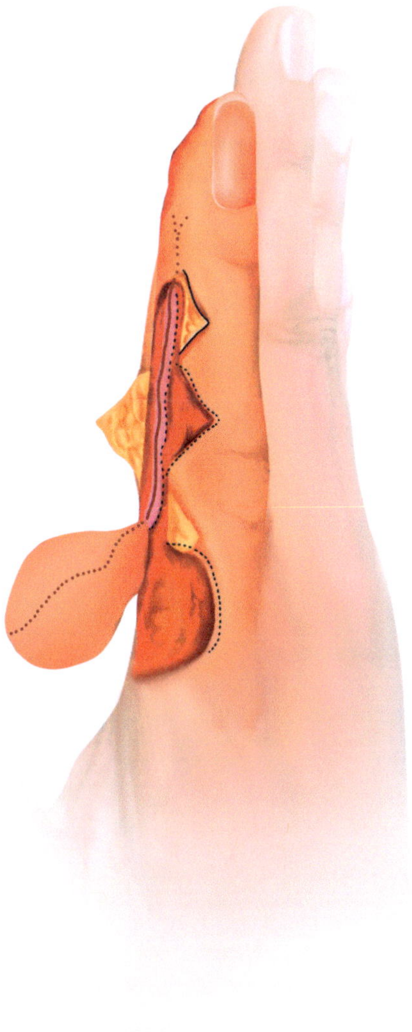

Fig. 22.1 The proposed flap design. The flap is marked centered over the digital artery on the dorsolateral aspect of the proximal phalanx after confirming digital vascular bundle patency with digital Allen's test. The flap is then raised in a proximal to distal fashion. The digital nerve is identified and separated from the digital artery. The flap is then raised after ligating the proximal digital artery and including the vessel in the flap as its pedicle. The flap is then rotated and inset to the fingertip defect

- After division, the flap can be rotated to 180 degrees to the defect area.
- Flap insetting is done using minimal loose sutures to avoid congestion in the postoperative period and have enough space to allow for postoperative swelling.
- The skin tail included in the flap design is used at the time of insetting to cover the area over the pedicle. If the skin tail is not included in the design, a skin graft can be applied to avoid constricting the area.
- The donor area is covered with FTSG and tie-over dressing is done.

Postop Care [1, 2]

- Noncircumferential soft dressing for the finger is done.
- Hand is elevated without a splint.
- Physical therapy can be started once flap vascularity is confirmed in the postop period, usually within the first week postoperatively.
- Scar management is then initiated after complete flap healing.

Complications [1, 7]

- Flap congestion.
- Partial flap loss.
- Complete flap loss.
- Flexion contracture at the PIPJ level.

Variants [7–10]

- Adipofascial flap.
- Neurovascular flap.
- Heterodigital cross-finger flap.
- Heterodigital flap.

References

1. Seah BZQ, Sebastin SJ, Chong AKS. Retrograde flow digital artery flaps. Hand Clin. 2020;36:47–56.
2. Lai CS, Lin SD, Yang CC. The reverse digital artery flap for fingertip reconstruction. Ann Plast Surg. 1989;22:495.
3. Han SK, Lee BL, Kim WK. The reverse digital artery island flap: clinical experience in 120 fingers. Plast Reconstr Surg. 1998;101:4.
4. Yazar M, Aydın A, Kurt Yazar S, et al. Sensory recovery of the reverse homodigital island flap in fingertip reconstruction: a review of 66 cases. Acta Orthop Traumatol Turc. 2010;44(5):345–51.
5. Lin B-J, Shih J-T, Le H-M. Clinical experience using a reverse homodigital island flap in nearby fingertip reconstruction. J Med Sci. 2007;27(3):109–12.
6. Buncke HJ, Rose HE. Free toe-to-fingertip neurovascular flaps. Plast Reconstr Surg. 1979;63:607.
7. Karacalar A, Sen C, Ozcan M. A modified reversed digital island flap incorporating the proper digital nerve. Ann Plast Surg. 2000;45(1):67–70.
8. Chang KP, Wang WH, Lai CS, et al. Refinement of reverse digital arterial flap for finger defects: surgical technique. J Hand Surg Am. 2005;30(3):558–61.
9. Lai CS, Lin SD, Tsai CC, et al. Reverse digital artery neurovascular cross-finger flap. J Hand Surg Am. 1995;20(3):397–402.
10. Adani R, Busa R, Scagni R, et al. The heterodigital reversed flow neurovascular island flap for fingertip injuries. J Hand Surg Br. 1999;24(4):431–6.

Quaba Flap

23

Ezekwe E. Amirize and Turki Alhassan

Classification [1–3] Island axial pattern (reverse-flow) flap.

Vascular Supply [1, 3–7]
- The Quaba perforator arises from the dorsal communicating branch of the common digital artery.
- The first, second, and third dorsal metacarpal arteries (DMAs) are present more than 95% of the time, whereas the fourth and fifth are more variable originating from the palmer system when the dorsal system is not present.
- The DMA system courses distally and anastomoses with the palmar system. At the junction of these two systems, there is a perforator that branches to supply the skin on the dorsum of the hand.
- This is the perforator from the dorsal communicating branch of the common digital artery, also known as the Quaba perforator.
- The flow through this perforator can be antegrade through the DMA or retrograde from the palmar system or the dorsal digital arteries.
- Venous drainage is conducted by venae comitantes of the perforator in a reverse fashion.

Innervation [1, 3] An insensate flap.

Indications [1, 3]
- Defects in the following areas of the hand:
  - Dorsum of the hand adjacent to the metacarpophalangeal joint (MCPJ).
  - Phalangeal skin dorsal defect, up to distal interphalangeal joint.

E. E. Amirize · T. Alhassan (✉)
Plastic Surgery Division, Department of Surgery, Ministry of National Guard - Health Affairs, King Abdullah International Medical Research Center, Riyadh, Saudi Arabia

O. Almeshal et al. (eds.), *Soft Tissue Reconstruction of the Hand: Loco-regional and Distant Flaps Selection and Approach*,
https://doi.org/10.1007/978-981-16-9945-0_23

- Interdigital webspaces.
- Distal palmar defects.

Contraindications [3, 6]

- Crush hand injuries.
- Local hand infections.
- Compromised vascular anatomy of the hand, such as from deep webspace laceration or fracture of meta-carpal head or neck.

Advantages [1, 6, 8, 9]

- One-stage procedure which allows for finger mobilization.
- Reliability and ease of raising the flap.
- Good color match, skin texture, etc., like other local flaps.
- Possibility of raising more than one flap in one hand to cover multiple defects.
- Feasible flap preexpansion for coverage of larger defects.
- Capacity to incorporate tendon graft in the flap.
- Possibility of modifying the flap to reach defects on middle and distal phalanx dorsum, such as the use of curved ellipse flap design or ligation and division of the DMA proximal to the perforator.
- Acceptable donor site morbidity.

Disadvantages [1, 6, 8, 9]

- Insensate flap (However, the flap is usually required to cover areas with crude sensation.).
- Donor sites greater than 2 cm wide not be closed primarily.
- Difficulty in reaching the distal palm and volar surface proximal phalanx (Flap tunneling to increase reach can compromise venous return).
- The hair-bearing skin of the hand dorsum not suitable for the palm and web spaces, especially in dark-skinned people, which should be avoided.

Marking Technique [1, 4, 7–9]

- A handheld Doppler is used to locate the Quaba perforator in the appropriate intermetacarpal space. This site is usually 0.5 cm to 1 cm proximal to the adjacent MCPJ. From here, the axis of flap rotation is marked (Fig. 23.1a).
- Adjacent to the dorsal hand defect, a longitudinal ellipse is marked, spanning from the MCPJ distally to the proximal wrist crease. The width is marked between 1 cm and 3.5 cm, with the outer lateral border of the adjoining metacarpal as the lateral limit.
- A curved ellipse flap design with a cutaneous bridge segment is a variation (Fig. 23.1b).
- Intraoperatively, the intertendinous connection is useful as a guide to the Quaba perforator.
- Flap is usually marked in the second, third, or fourth inter-metacarpal spaces.
- The perforator is present constantly in the second and third space.

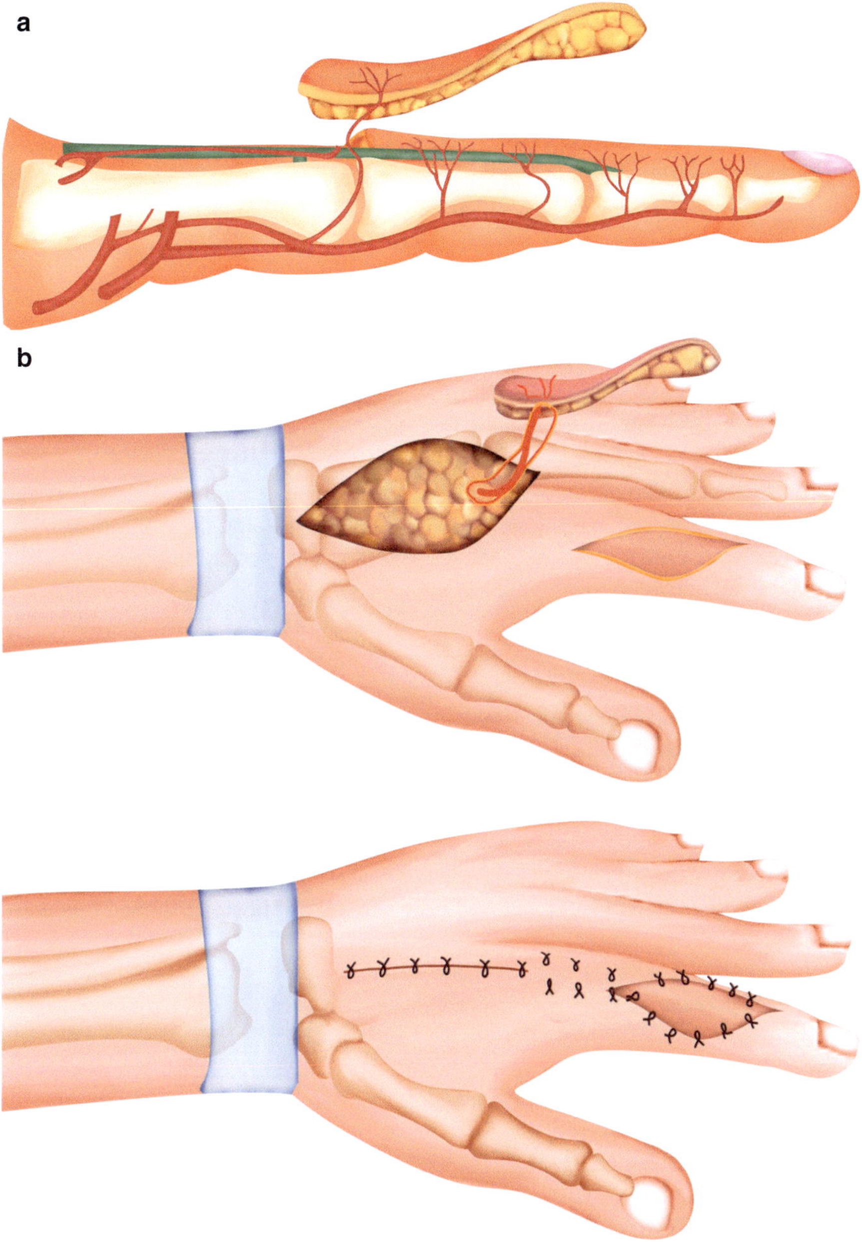

Fig. 23.1 (**a**) The location of the flap perforator in the inter-metacarpal space (second, third, or fourth intermetacarpal spaces). This is usually 0.5 cm to 1 cm proximal to the adjacent metacarpo-phalangeal joint. From this point, the axis of flap rotation is also marked. (**b**) The proposed flap design and its rotation. A dorsal hand ellipse that is based on the marked perforator is designed

The flap is then raised in a proximal to distal fashion. When reaching near the marked perforator, the extensor tendons are then retracted to visualize the perforator better. The perforating vessel is usually seen immediately distal to the juncturae. The flap is then rotated to the defect, and the donor site is closed primarily.

Surgical Technique [1, 3, 4, 8]

- Under general anesthesia, the patient is lying supine with hand on arm table; flap marking is done.
- Tourniquet is applied.
- Defect is debrided and hemostasis secured.
- The tourniquet is inflated, avoiding exsanguination for easy pedicle identification.
- Using microsurgical loupe, the flap is elevated proximally to distally.
- From one side of the marked ellipse, a skin incision is made and carried down just superficial to the extensor paratenon.
- Proximally, the flap elevation begins with gentle undermining.
- As dissection approaches the site marked for the perforator, the extensor tendons are retracted to visualize the perforator better. The perforating vessel is seen immediately distal to the juncturae.
- As the perforator is identified, the flap length and its axis of rotation are confirmed.
- Next, the incision is made on the contralateral side of the ellipse and dissection is carried out as described.
- Superficial veins are ligated, converting the flap to an island.
- The flap pedicle is not skeletonized.
- The tourniquet is released, flap viability is checked, and hemostasis is secured.
- The flap is then rotated within an arc of 0–180° to cover the defect.
- Further dissection of the pedicle into the inter-metacarpal space and dividing the DMA proximally allow flap coverage of distal palmer defects.
- The flap donor defect can be closed primarily in two layers if its width is 2 cm or less.
- Occasionally, if a larger flap was harvested or if there is significant hand swelling, the secondary defect is skin-grafted.

Postop Care [3, 8]

- Fingers and wrist mobilized in extension.
- Hand ROM exercises initiated in 1 week if skin graft was not used in the reconstruction.
- Ten days of hand immobilization if donor defect was skin-grafted.

Variants

- Maruyama flap [5, 8, 10]:
  - It is a similar skin island to the Quaba flap; however, all soft tissues between the extensor tendons and deep fascia over dorsal interosseous muscle are taken.
  - The main DMA is divided.
  - It is raised on all five DMAs.

- Reconstructing extensor tendons at recipient sites (e.g., a central slip) [1]:
  - Quaba flap can be raised with a vascularized extensor digitorum communis tendon graft, for example, in soft tissue defects associated with Boutonniere deformity, as seen in burn rheumatoid arthritis of the hand.
- Covering multiple defects [1]:
  - More than one Quaba flap can be raised in the same hand.
- Preexpanded flap [1]:
  - With a tissue expander placed in a pocket in proximal two-thirds of the hand (to avoid damage to the perforator), the Quaba flap can be preexpanded.
- Flap design as a curved ellipse [8, 9]:
  - This offers an additional 0.8–1.0 cm of length at the flap inset, more than the straight ellipse.

Case

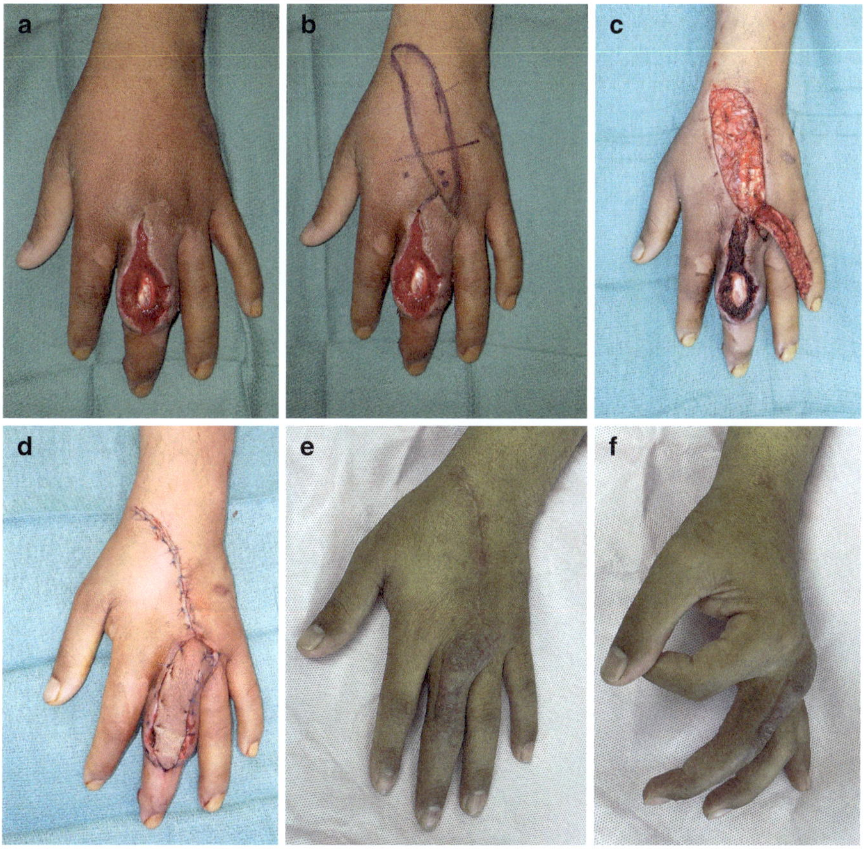

Case 23.1 Intraoperative photo of a patient who presented with post-debridement wound over the dorsum of middle finger with exposed extensor tendons in (**a**). After ensuring good wound irrigation, coverage was planned with Quaba flap as it was marked over the third intermetacarpal spaces as shown in (**b**). Flap perforator was marked with the help of handheld Doppler ultrasound. The flap was then elevation, ensuring intact intermetacarpal perforator as seen in (**c**). The flap was then rotated and inset to cover the defect as seen in (**d**). Follow assessment of the patient five months after the procedure is shown in (**e**) and (**f**)

References

1. Quaba AA, Davidson PM. The distally-based dorsal hand flap. Br J Plast Surg. 1990;43:28–39.
2. Cormack GC, Lamberty BGH. A classification of fasciocutaneous flaps according to their patterns of vascularization. Br J Plast Surg. 1984;37:80–7.
3. Al-Baz TH, Gad SS, Keshk TF, Aly MS. Evaluation of dorsal metacarpal artery perforator flaps in the reconstruction of hand soft tissue defects. Menoufia Med J. 2019;32(4):1256–61.
4. Martinez FM, MLG N, Navarro JG, Ros AG, Robledano AI. Hand coverage. In: Amr S, editor. Issues in flap surgery. InTech; 2018.
5. Masson JA. Hand I: finger nails, infections, tumours and soft-tissue reconstruction. In Selected readings in plastic surgery, Vol 9, No. 32; 2002.
6. Omokawa S, et al. The anatomical basis for reverse first to fifth dorsal metacarpal arterial flaps. J Hand Surg Br. 2005;30(1):40–4.
7. Bailey SH, Andry D, Saint-Cyr M. The dorsal metacarpal artery perforator flap: a case report utilizing a quaba flap harvested from a previously skin-grafted area for dorsal 5th digit coverage. Hand (N Y). 2010;5(3):322–5.
8. Rehim SA, Chung KC. Local flaps of the hand. Hand Clin. 2014;30:137–51.
9. Chung KC, Moran SL. ASSH surgical anatomy: flap reconstruction; 2019.
10. Maruyama Y. The reverse dorsal metacarpal flap. Br J Plast Surg. 1990;43:24–7.

Part IV

Thumb-Related Flaps

Moberg Volar Advancement Flap

24

Anas M. Alyamani and Abdulaziz Alhujayri

Classification [1] Local axial fasciocutaneous advancement flap of the thumb.

Vascular Supply [1] The Moberg flap is a bipedicled flap of the thumb based on both digital arteries.

Innervation [1] Both digital nerves are included to provide sensation to the flap.

Indications [2–4]

- Moberg flap is a well-known flap to cover defects of the thumb pulp. The defect size that can be covered varies in the literature from 1.8 to 3 cm in longitudinal (proximal to distal) diameter.
- Snow has also described this flap for the tip of the index defect due to the similar dual vascularity.
- Macht published a series of using this flap for the other digit by ensuring the preservation of the dorsal perforators to preserve the dorsal supply.

Contraindications

- Injury to the digital arteries of the thumb or the princeps pollicis artery.
- Young patients who require dexterous motion in the hand (artist, pianist, etc.).

Advantages [5]

- Near-normal sensation.
- Easy to perform and advance.
- Ideal for volar thumb defects.

A. M. Alyamani · A. Alhujayri (✉)
Plastic Surgery Division, Department of Surgery, Ministry of National Guard - Health Affairs, King Abdullah International Medical Research Center, Riyadh, Saudi Arabia

O. Almeshal et al. (eds.), *Soft Tissue Reconstruction of the Hand: Loco-regional and Distant Flaps Selection and Approach*,
https://doi.org/10.1007/978-981-16-9945-0_24

Disadvantages

- Risk of IP joint stiffness.
- Hyperesthesia.
- Cold intolerance.
- Jeopardizing other options for thumb reconstruction.

Marking Technique [6]

- The flap is marked along the mid-axial lines of the thumb. The proximal edge of the flap corresponds with the level of flexion crease of the MCP joint (Fig. 24.1).

Surgical Technique

- At the distal end of the flap, a full-thickness skin incision is made along the mid-axial lines.
- The flap is dissected off the flexor pollicis longus tendon incorporating digital vessels and nerves.
- Once the flap is freed from all but its proximal attachment, it can be advanced toward the distal end and sutured to the tip of the thumb to cover the defect.
- Donor site defect is usually covered with a skin graft.

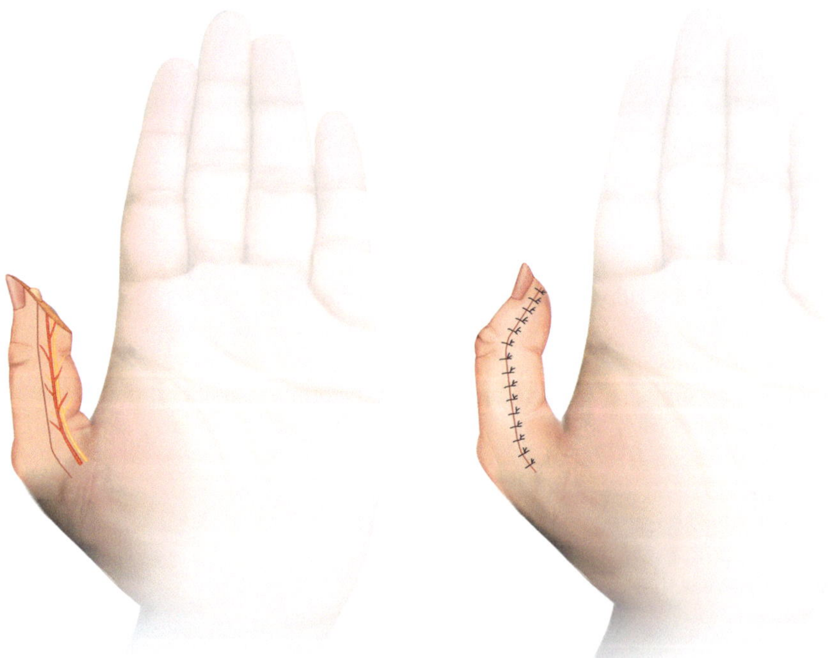

Fig. 24.1 The proposed flap design. The flap is designed and marked along the mid-axial lines of the thumb ending proximally at the level of flexion crease of the MCP joint. After the flap is dissected off the flexor tendon sheath, the flap is raised, including the volar neurovascular bundles. The flap is then mobilized and with the aid of interphalangeal joint flexion, the flap is inset to cover the thumb tip defect

Postop Care [6]

- No standard immobilization regimen for postoperative care: Posner and Smith applied a cast for 3 weeks and O'Brien preferred 10 days of immobilization.

Complications [4]

- The most common complaints are pain and cold sensitivity.

Variants [7–9]

- Dellon's modification of flap design into the webspace increases advancement to 3.0 cm.
- O'Brien made a proximal transverse incision along the MCP joint crease; again, this converts the flap into an island flap.
- Elliot modified the O'Brien advancement flap. The proximal portion of the flap is designed in a V fashion, extending proximally to the thenar eminence. This then allows V-Y closure of the base of the defect without an additional skin graft or lateral transposition flaps.

Case

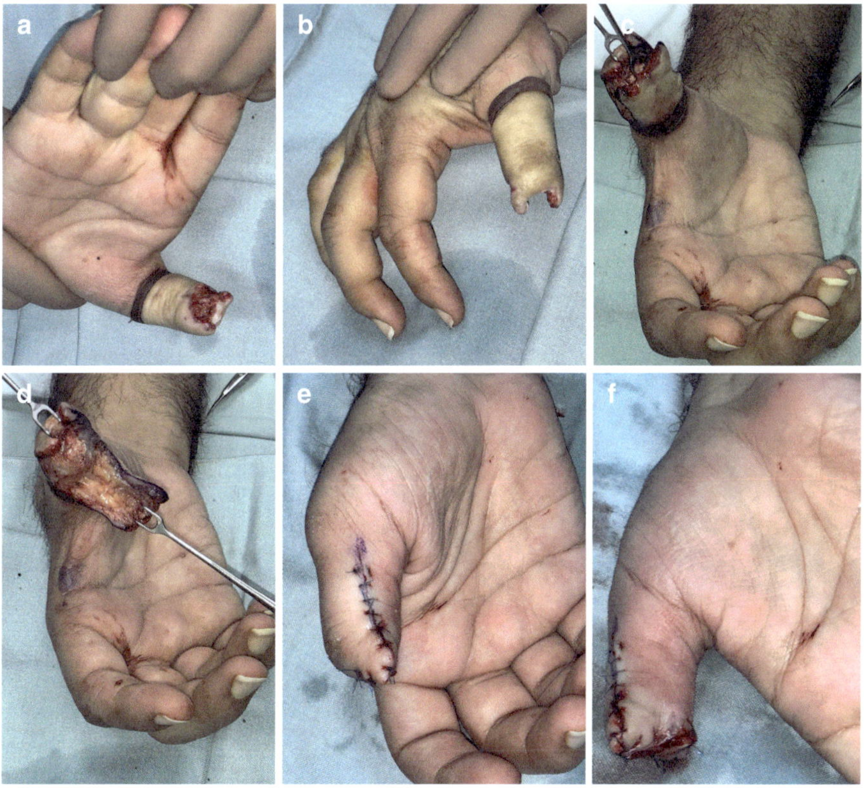

Case 24.1 Intraoperative photo of a patient who presented with traumatic thumb amputation with exposed distal phalanx as shown in (**a**) and (**b**). After good wound irrigation, coverage was planned with Moberg volar advancement flap as seen (**c**). The flap was elevated on top of the flexor sheath as seen (**d**). Flap was advanced and inset to cover the distal thumb defect with slight bend of the distal interphalangeal joint as shown in (**e**) and (**f**)

References

1. Wink JD, et al. Flap reconstruction of the hand. Plast Reconstruct Surg. 2020;145(1):172e–83e.
2. Baumeister S, et al. Functional outcome after the Moberg advancement flap in the thumb. J Hand Surg. 2002;27(1):105–14.
3. Snow JW. The use of a volar flap for repair of fingertip amputations; A preliminary report. Plast Reconstr Surg. 1967;40:163.
4. Macht SD, Watson HK. The Moberg volar advancement flap for digital reconstruction. J Hand Surg. 1980;5(4):372–6.
5. Foucher G, et al. Long-term outcome of neurovascular palmar advancement flaps for distal thumb injuries. Br J Plast Surg. 1999;52(1):64–8.
6. Rehim SA, Chung KC. Local flaps of the hand. Hand Clin. 2014;30(2):137–51, v.
7. Dellon AL. The extended palmar advancement flap. J Hand Surg. 1983;8(2):190–4.
8. O'Brien B. Neurovascular island pedicle flaps for terminal amputations and digital scars. Br J Plast Surg. 1968;21(3):258–61.
9. Elliot D, Wilson Y. V-Y advancement of the entire volar soft tissue of the thumb in distal reconstruction. J Hand Surg (Edinburgh, Scotland). 1993;18(3):399–402.

25 Neurovascular Island Pedicled (Littler) Flap

Asmaa Z. Bin Mahmoud and Abdulaziz Alhujayri

Classification [1, 2] Innervated axial pattern regional flap (interpolation)

Vascular Supply Ulnar digital artery, either the 3rd or the 4th digit

Innervation Ulnar digital nerve, either the 3rd or the 4th digit

Indications [1, 2]
- Scarred, tender thumb pulp, with decreased sensation and/or ischemic tip.
- Historically and recently with some modifications, to restore the sensation of the thumb in unrepairable median nerve injury.

Contraindications [1]
- Jeopardizing blood supply to middle or ring fingers.
- Anomaly in the palmar arch vascular tree.

Advantages [1, 3]
- Bringing sensate pliable and vascularized soft tissue to cover distal thumb defect.
- Long vascular pedicle when ulnar digital artery of the middle finger is used.

Disadvantages [1, 3]
- Sacrificing ulnar-sided sensation of other digits (Some are elected to reconstruct the nerve with a nerve graft.).
- Insufficient venous drainage due to small veins.

A. Z. B. Mahmoud · A. Alhujayri (✉)
Plastic Surgery Division, Department of Surgery, Ministry of National Guard - Health Affairs, King Abdullah International Medical Research Center, Riyadh, Saudi Arabia

O. Almeshal et al. (eds.), *Soft Tissue Reconstruction of the Hand: Loco-regional and Distant Flaps Selection and Approach*,
https://doi.org/10.1007/978-981-16-9945-0_25

- Incomplete sensory recovery of the thumb, as the brain still processes the input as if coming from donor digit.
- Delicate dissection of the neurovascular bundle, especially proximally, to provide sufficient length for interpolation.

Marking Technique [1, 3]

- The donor digit is chosen based on intact innervation: if median nerve is intact, the flap is from the ulnar third digit; if the median nerve is not intact and ulnar nerve is intact, the flap is from the ulnar side of fourth digit (Fig. 25.1).
- The primary defect is measured and modeled.
- The template is applied over the ulnar aspect of the middle or ring digits. The flap can be extended as far as the webspace and beyond the tip of donor digit.
- Palmar incision is designed as zigzag incision ends just proximal to the flexor retinaculum.

Surgical Technique [1]

- Handheld Doppler is used to assess hand circulation and both vessels for the proposed donor digit and the ulnar side of the adjacent digit.

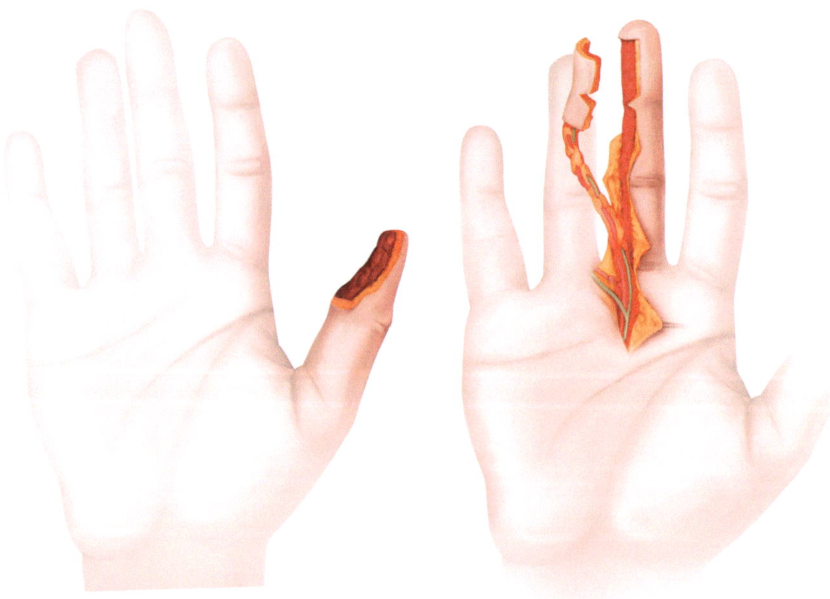

Fig. 25.1 The proposed flap design. The flap is marked on the ulnar aspect of the ulnar side of the middle finger on the distal phalanx. That is based on the template of the thumb defect. A Bruner's zigzag incision type is created to dissect freely the digital neurovascular bundle that is the flap pedicle. The dissection is carried out till the palm. The radial digital artery to the ring finger is then identified and ligated. The proper digital nerves to the third webspace are traced and dissected with interfascicular dissection to separate the nerves further. The flap is then mobilized and tunneled subcutaneously to the thumb defect

- Thorough debridement and irrigation of the thumb defect are done; then, the primary defect is measured and a template is created.
- If the thumb digital nerve is anastomosed to the transferred digital nerve, it is advised to use the ulnar digital nerve of the thumb. However, if not intended to be used, the nerve is dissected more proximally and transected at the muscle belly level to avoid painful neuroma.
- The template is applied over the ulnar aspect of the middle or ring digits.
- The tourniquet is elevated.
- Initial dissection is carried out at the palmar level to ensure normal vascular territory. If the initial dissection within the palm showed abnormal vascular tree, the procedure should be shifted toward other options for coverage.
- Once the vascular tree is identified as normal, dissection can be started on the finger.
- Palmar skin and subcutaneous tissues are incised to the flexor sheath, and dissection dorsally is carried out via blunt scissors till reaching the dorsal incision.
- With gentle dorsal traction of the flap, the small branches to the flexor sheath and interphalangeal joints are visualized and divided and dissection proceeds to proximal direction.
- It is essential to keep the pedicle as a monobloc of fatty tissue throughout the dissection process, which will enhance venous drainage.
- The radial digital artery to the ring finger and the communicating branch from the metacarpal artery are identified and ligated.
- Then, the proper digital nerves to the third web space are traced and dissected, to split them from each other.
- Once the palmar arch is visualized, dissection should stop.
- A subcutaneous tunnel is created via blunt scissors, just superficial to palmar fascia, wide enough to pass the blunt scissors with opened tips.
- It is immensely important to study the relationship between the radial digital nerve of the ring finger and ulnar digital artery of the middle finger at the palmar arch level, as it is not uncommon that a close relationship causes kinking once the pedicle is passed to the thumb. The entire pedicle should pass underneath the intact fourth radial digital nerve to overcome this potential problem.
- A 1-inch Penrose drain is passed from the 1ry defect to pass the flap, through the tunnel till the palmar incision; then, a stay suture is fixed into flap tip and handled to the hemostat which is inside the Penrose. Once the suture is handled, the flap is slowly withdrawn till it reaches the 1ry defect and then the Penrose can be removed.
- The flap is secured with one stitch and the thumb should be kept in full abduction and extension at all times and checked for any tension or kink, and if none, proceed with flap inset with nonabsorbable sutures as one layer.
- The tourniquet is released, the viability of the flap is checked, and hemostasis is secured.
- A shin graft is applied to the donor site and secured with tie-over dressing.
- Apply noncircumferential dressing and full cast with thumb spica.
- Keep window for flap monitoring.

Postop Care [1]

- Dressing is kept intact till the primary dressing change of the graft.
- The viability of the flap is checked, and a few marginal stitches are removed if the flow is insufficient.
- Thumb movement is allowed at 3–4 weeks postoperatively.

Complications

- Partial or complete flap necrosis.
- Stiffness of the donor digit.
- Venous congestion.

Variants [4, 5]

- Twin neurovascular island flap, from the radial aspect of ring finger and ulnar aspect of middle finger.
- Harvesting both proper digital nerve and dorsal digital nerve of the donor site to ensure proper restoration of the sensation.

References

1. Green's operative hand surgery, 6th and 7th edition.
2. Littler JW. The neurovascular pedicle method of digital trans-position for reconstruction of the thumb. Plast Reconstr Surg. 1953;12:303–19.
3. Chao, et al. Local hand flaps. J Am Soc Surg Hand. 2001;1(1).
4. Chen H, Noordhoff S. Coverage of the degloved thumb with twin neurovascular island flaps: a case report. Br J Plas Surg. 1986;39:255–6.
5. Wang H, Yang X, Chen C, Wang B, Wang W, Jia S. Modified Littler flap for sensory reconstruction of large thumb pulp defects. J Hand Surg (Eur Vol). 2018;43(5):546–53.

Annular Flap

26

Asmaa Z. Bin Mahmoud and Abdulaziz Alhujayri

Classification [1] Tetra-pedicled homodigital island flap

Vascular Supply Radial and ulnar digital arteries of the thumb

Innervation [1] Radial and ulnar digital nerves of the thumb

Indication
- When senate flap is required for distal thumb defect.

Contraindications
- Disruption to one or both neurovascular bundles.

Advantages
- Restoring the sensation at the distal aspect of the thumb.
- Reliable option with intact neurovascular bundle.

Disadvantages
- Limited mobility to cover the distal wounds.
- Delicate dissection of the neurovascular bundles.
- Scaring and contracture at the donor site.

Marking Technique [1]
- A circular line is marked 2 cm proximal to the defect at the tip of the finger (Fig. 26.1).

A. Z. Bin Mahmoud · A. Alhujayri (✉)
Plastic Surgery Division, Department of Surgery, Ministry of National Guard - Health Affairs, King Abdullah International Medical Research Center, Riyadh, Saudi Arabia

O. Almeshal et al. (eds.), *Soft Tissue Reconstruction of the Hand: Loco-regional and Distant Flaps Selection and Approach*,
https://doi.org/10.1007/978-981-16-9945-0_26

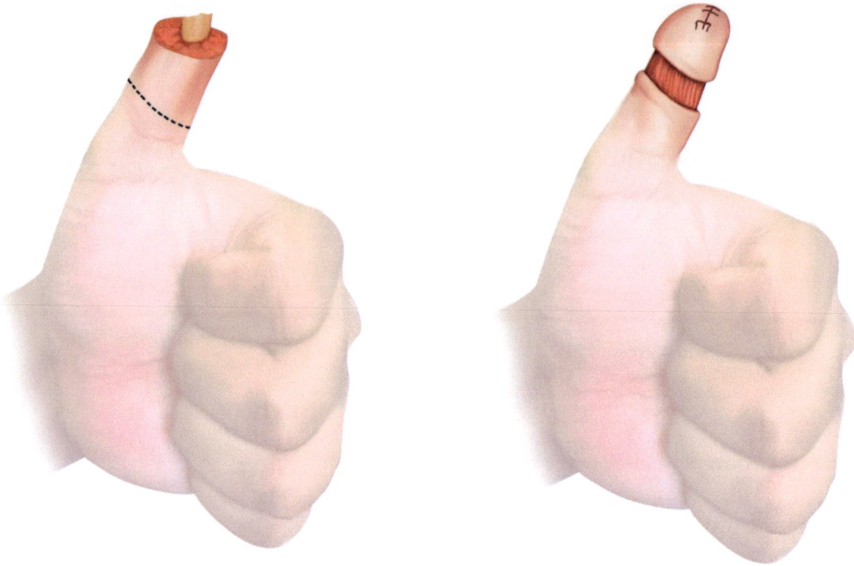

Fig. 26.1 The proposed flap marking site on the thumb. The flap is marked as a circular incision around the finger that is about 2 cm proximal to the defect on the fingertip. The incision is then created, and dissection is made over only to the subcutaneous tissue where the neurovascular bundles are dissected longitudinally to allow flap mobilization and maintained intact. The flap is then mobilized distally, and the donor site is skin grafted

Surgical Technique [1, 3]

- After marking the circular incision, 2 cm proximal to the skin defect, only the skin and the subcutaneous tissue are incised.
- Both neurovascular bundles are identified and dissected proximally and distally to allow free mobility of tissues, almost 10–12 mm.
- The distal aspect is approximated in a tension-free manner with a single layer of sutures. If the closure is tight, it can be allowed to heal by secondary intention.
- The primary defect is either grafted or left to heal via secondary intention.
- Noncircumferential loose dressing with paraffin gauze, then povidone-soaked dressing, and then thumb spica splint are used.

Postop Care

- The flap should be exposed for monitoring. The dressing is usually changed at the time of primary dressing of the skin graft if used.

Complications [3]

- Hyperesthesia.
- Venous congestion.
- Partial skin necrosis.

Variants None.

References

1. Chao, et al. Local hand flaps. J Am Soc Surg Hand. 2001;1(1).
2. Goumain AJ, Baudet J, Massard JF. Our experience with recent thumb mutilations. Revue de Chirurgie Orthopedique et Reparatrice de l'Appareil Moteur. 1972;58:563–74.
3. Handbook on flaps in crush injuries of the hand. New Delhi: Jaycee Brothers Medical Publisher; 2015.

First Dorsal Metacarpal Artery Flap and Its Variants (Foucher's Kite, Helovich's Racquet Flap, and Bilobed First Dorsal Metacarpal Artery Flap)

27

Asmaa Z. Bin Mahmoud and Abdulaziz Alhujayri

Classification [1] Axial pattern, island flap

Vascular Supply [2] First dorsal metacarpal artery (FDMA), a branch from the radial artery

Innervation [3] Branches from superficial radial nerve and dorsal branches from the index digital nerve

Indications [3]
- Soft tissue loss of palmar or dorsal aspects of distal thumb.
- To restore distal thumb sensation.
- To treat cold intolerance of the thumb.
- To overcome venous congestion after thumb replantation.

Contraindications [4]
- Active thumb infection.
- Trauma to the index finger that affected the arterial territory.
- Absence of preoperative Doppler signal.

A. Z. B. Mahmoud · A. Alhujayri (✉)
Plastic Surgery Division, Department of Surgery, Ministry of National Guard - Health Affairs, King Abdullah International Medical Research Center, Riyadh, Saudi Arabia

O. Almeshal et al. (eds.), *Soft Tissue Reconstruction of the Hand: Loco-regional and Distant Flaps Selection and Approach*,
https://doi.org/10.1007/978-981-16-9945-0_27

Advantages
- Consistent anatomical location of the first metacarpal artery.
- Easy to harvest and transpose.

Disadvantages [4, 6]
- Absence of cortical representation.
- 2PD of 9–10 mm

Marking of Foucher's Flap [3, 5]
- The defect is modeled by creating a template (Fig. 27.1).

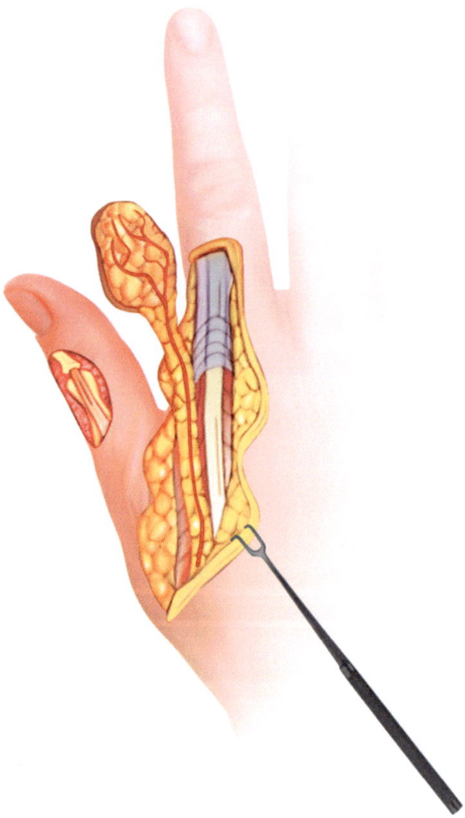

Fig. 27.1 The dissected and raised first dorsal metacarpal artery flap. The course of the artery was mapped with handheld Doppler ultrasound. The flap was marked on the dorsal surface of the index proximal phalanx. The flap was then elevated over the extensor tendon paratenon. Proximally, the dorsal longitudinal lazy S incision was done to dissect the pedicle further. The pedicle enters the flap at the radial aspect of the index metacarpophalangeal joint. The dissection is deepened to include the extensor hood as the vessel is included in it. Subperiosteal dissection of the second metacarpal bone is done on the ulnar side and to the first dorsal interosseous muscle fascia radially. Dissection is done till enough pedicle length is reached. After which, the flap is tunneled to the thumb defect, and the donor site is skin grafted

- The distal limit of the flap is the index proximal interphalangeal joint, and the proximal limit is the second metacarpophalangeal joint.
- A lazy "S" incision is drawn parallel to the radial border of the second metacarpal bone.

Surgical Technique of Foucher's Flap [2, 5]

- The course of FDMA is mapped with handheld Doppler, from the radial aspect of the index MPJ till the pivot point.
- Thorough debridement of the thumb is commenced; then, a template of the defect is created.
- The pattern is transposed over the dorsum of the index proximal phalanx.
- The tourniquet is elevated.
- The ulnar aspect of the flap is incised.
- Move along the loose areolar plane, just above the extensor tendon paratenon, and proceed from the proximal to distal direction.
- Care should be taken when it comes to the radial aspect of index MPJ, where the FDMA enters the flap content.
- At this level, the level of dissection is deepened to include part of the extensor hood to make sure that the vessel is included within the flap.
- The second metacarpal bone is identified ulnarly, the periosteum incised, and the dissection carried out radially deep to the first dorsal interosseous muscle fascia.
- The pedicle is dissected by incising the radial aspect of the first interosseous muscle and the ulnar aspect of second metacarpal bone.
- Dorsal veins and branches from the radial sensory nerve join the flap from the ulnar aspect of the index MPJ, and they are identified and included within the flap.
- The pedicle is then dissected proximally till the pivot point at the base of the first and second metacarpals.
- The tourniquet is released and hemostasis is secured.
- A wide subcutaneous tunnel is created, with a teardrop design to the flap, which allows for tension-free closure.
- The flap is tagged at the recipient site with a suture, and the tourniquet is released to ensure flap viability and secure hemostasis.
- Flap is secured with nonabsorbable sutures.
- The index donor site and third digit in bilobed flap are skin grafted and secured with tie-over dressing.
- Noncircumferential nonadherent dressing is applied with a window to monitor the flap, and full-cast thumb spica is used.

Postop Care [5]

- Dressing is kept intact till primary dressing change of the graft.
- The viability of the flap is checked, and a few marginal stitches are removed if the flow is insufficient.

Complications [4, 6]

- Decreased ROM of thumb interphalangeal joint, around 15 degrees.
- Higher rates of venous congestion and partial flap necrosis in island flaps (Foucher's design).
- Higher rates of cold intolerance in island flaps when compared to racquet flap [6].
- Decreased protective sensation of index and mild decrease in ROM.

Variants [3]

- *Racquet flap*: it is the same as an island flap; however, it includes skin over the pedicle and no subcutaneous tunnel. A dorsal incision is created over the desired path on the thumb.
- *Bilobed flap*: it is considered as a salvage procedure after failed thumb replantation or degloving injury. It includes both first and second metacarpal arteries. After mapping first and second DMA, the dissection started ulnarly over the dorsum of the middle finger proximal phalanx with a small cut in the connecting skin between the third and second digits. The dissection is superficial to the extensor paratenon. Proximally, a lazy "S" incision is made if a fascial pedicle is desired or a longitudinal skin design is created to include skin as in racquet flap.

Case

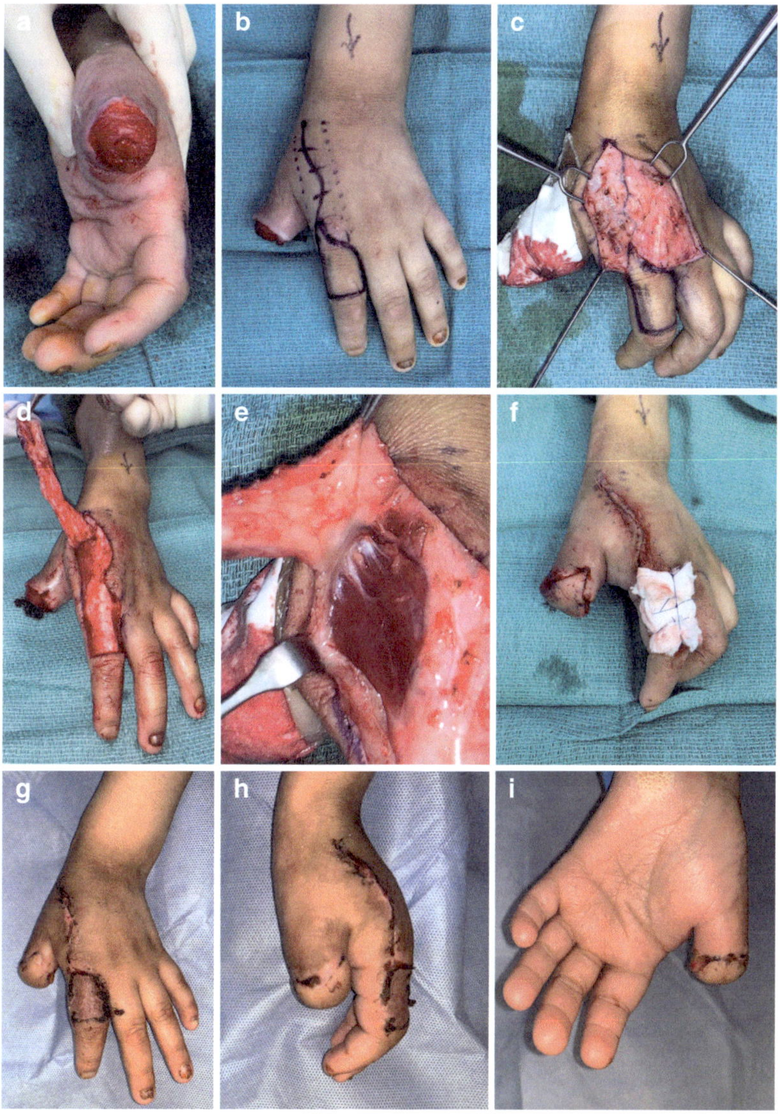

Case 27.1 Intraoperative photo of a patient who acquired a traumatic amputation of the thumb proximal to the interphalangeal joint with exposed bone as shown in (**a**) Coverage was planned with pedicled first dorsal metacarpal artery flap that was marked as shown in (**b**) over the dorsum of index proximal phalanx with prober reverse planning to ensure flap reach. The skin incision was first made over the dorsum of the index metacarpal area with care for the dorsal veins and adipofascial tissue as seen in (**c**). Then, dissection proceeded after identification of the second metacarpal bone ulnarly, in which the periosteum is incised, and the dissection carried out radially deep to the 1st dorsal interosseous muscle fascia. The pedicle is then dissected proximally till the pivot point at the base of the first and second metacarpals as seen (**d**) and (**e**). Flap was then moved to the defect after ensuring wide subcutaneous tunnel to avoid any compression on the tunneled pedicle and the donor site was skin grafted as seen (**f**). Follow-up assessment at 1-month postop is shown in (**g**), (**h**), and (**i**) with good soft tissue coverage

References

1. Chao, et al. Local hand flaps. J Am Soc Surg Hand. 2001;1(1).
2. Rahim SA, Chung KC. Local flaps of the hand. Hand Clin. 2014;30:137–51.
3. Couceiro J, de Prado M, Menendez G, Manteiga Z. First dorsal metacarpal artery flap family: a review. Surg J. 2018;4:e215–9.
4. Prabhu M, Power R, Sulhyan SR. FDMA flap: a versatile technique to reconstruct the thumb. Int J Pharm Med Bio Sci. 2013.
5. Green's operative hand surgery, 7th edition.
6. Couceriro J, Sanmartin M. The Holevich flap revisited: a comparison with the Foucher flap, case series. Hand Surg. 2014;19(3):469–74.

Reverse Dorsoradial "Moschella" Flap

28

Bushra Alhazmi and Abdulaziz Alhujayri

Classification [1] Axial pattern flap, a retrograde homodigital unipedicled skin flap

Vascular Supply [2] Dorsoradial collateral artery, originating from the radial artery

Innervation [1] Superficial sensory radial nerve branch, if the neural anastomosis is attempted

Indications [1, 3]
- Soft tissue defect of palmar or dorsal aspects of distal thumb.
- Soft tissue defect of the radial aspect overlying the proximal or distal phalanx of the thumb.

Contraindications [3, 4]
- Injury or thrombosis of the radial artery or the dorsoradial collateral artery.
- Injury of the donor area and close proximity of the zone of in- jury.
- Extensive scarring of the donor site.

Advantages [1, 5]
- One-stage procedure.
- Relatively simple procedure.
- Homodigital flap (especially useful in cases of mutilating hand trauma where utilizing other digits is not an option).
- Not sacrificing an important vascular structure such as the main radial artery.

B. Alhazmi · A. Alhujayri (✉)
Plastic Surgery Division, Department of Surgery, Ministry of National Guard - Health Affairs, King Abdullah International Medical Research Center, Riyadh, Saudi Arabia

O. Almeshal et al. (eds.), *Soft Tissue Reconstruction of the Hand: Loco-regional and Distant Flaps Selection and Approach*,
https://doi.org/10.1007/978-981-16-9945-0_28

- Providing thin and elastic flap that easily reaches the distal volar/dorsal aspects of the thumb.
- Limited hair growth over the donor site, if any, compared to other local options.
- Minimal donor site morbidity.
- Possibility of primary closure of the donor site resulting in esthetically acceptable scarring.
- Uncomplicated postoperative care that does not require immobilization of the unaffected digits.

Disadvantages [1, 5–7]

- Controversy exists regarding the anatomical consistency of the dorsoradial collateral artery.
- Flap transfer requires the division and inclusion of one of the branches of the superficial sensory radial nerve due to its proximity to the vascular axis.
- Average 2PD ranges from 9.4 to 10.63 mm in the literature. Sun et al. demonstrated that when flaps are inserted into the defect without performing neurorrhaphy, better sensory recovery was achieved with a small-sized flap.

Marking Technique [2, 3, 5]

- Using Doppler, the course of the dorsal radial digital artery is outlined, extending from its origin at the snuffbox to the middle point of the proximal phalanx, where anastomosis with the palmar vessels occurs.
- The artery travels at a mean distance of 1 cm from the median axis of the thumb (Fig. 28.1).
- The pivot point of the flap is marked that is the middle point of the proximal phalanx.

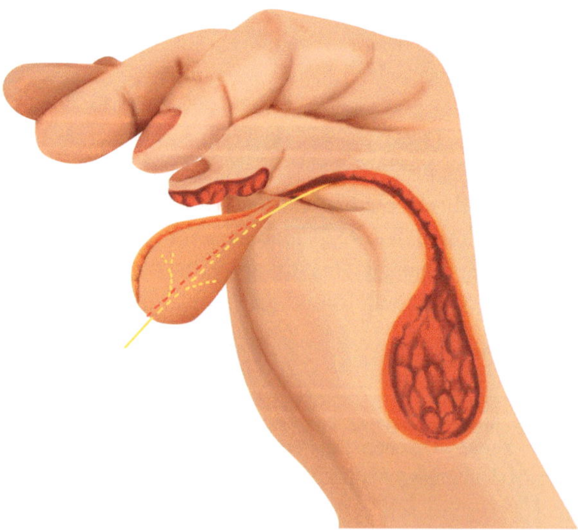

Fig. 28.1 The proposed flap harvest site. The flap is centered over the dorsal radial digital artery that extends from the snuffbox to the middle proximal phalanx, where its anastomosis with the palmar vessels occurs (The pivot point). The flap is rotated to cover the defect, and the donor site is primarily closed

- The skin island is drawn on the dorsal radial side of the first metacarpal, slightly larger than the defect size (20% oversize [6]), and is centered on the arterial axis. The shape can be tailored to the shape of the defect.
- The pedicle length is designed to be 3–4 mm longer than the distance calculated from the pivot point to the most proximal part of the defect to minimize the risk of vessel kinking.

Surgical Technique [1, 5]

- The procedure can be done under locoregional anesthesia with tourniquet control.
- Preparation and debridement of the recipient site are done initially.
- Skin incision is started at the distal edge of the flap, being very superficial to preserve the feeding vessel.
- The flap is raised in a plane just superficial to the paratenon in a proximal to distal dissection.
- The EPB tendon can be gently spread apart when encountered while elevating the flap.
- Then, the dorsal sensory nerve is identified. Because the nerve lies in very close proximity to the nutrient artery, it should be divided and bury the proximal stump while the distal end of the nerve is included within the flap.
- A zigzag or lazy "S" skin incision is made to harvest the pedicle. Then, a subcutaneous pedicle is raised with a considerable amount of loose tissue to protect the arterial axis and allow venous outflow. Isolating the vascular axis should not be attempted.
- Qin et al. showed that the designed pedicle's width from 0.6 to 0.8 cm yields significantly better outcomes compared to wider pedicles (up to 1.1 cm) in terms of esthetic patient satisfaction and time to return to work with no significant difference in venous congestion rate. The authors hypothesized that the venous network in a pedicle with a width of 0.6–0.8 cm is sufficient for venous drainage.
- Dissection of the pedicle is carried out along the thumb middle axis, starting from the distal edge of the flap and ending near the pivot point to protect the anastomosis with the palmar arterial circuit.
- Residual skin is incised between the pivot point and the defect if present.
- Tunneling the flap is avoided to decrease the risk of venous congestion.
- After completing the dissection and rotating the flap to the defect area, the tourniquet is deflated, and the perfusion with the flap in its original position is assessed.
- Provided that the flap is well perfused, hemostasis is secured, and the flap is reflected to the defect area.
- If neurorrhaphy is attempted, the dorsal radial nerve enclosed within the flap can be coapted to the stump of the volar digital nerve identified at the recipient site. Note that flap reinnervation has not been shown to have a superior sensory recovery.
- The flap is secured in place with loose sutures.

- The pedicle should not be under tension: if tension-free primary closure is difficult, leaving a small open area of the pedicle or closure with a skin bridge or a skin graft can be done.
- Donor defect is closed primarily in a tension-free fashion or by placing an FTSG.

Postop Care [1]
- Monitoring flap color and capillary refill.
- Thumb immobilization for 12–14 days and hand elevation.
- Starting active mobilization of the digit 2 weeks postoperatively, provided that no other procedures were performed.

Complications [1]
- Venous congestion.
- Partial flap loss.
- Mild decrease in ROM of the IPJ (by few degrees only, which might be attributed to the initial associated soft tissue/bony injuries) [7].
- Mild cold intolerance of the flap [7].
- Mild pain or hypersensitivity on the flap [7].
- Mild pain on the donor site [7].

Variants
- Cross-finger flap: [8] the use of the reverse dorsoradial skin flap to reconstruct the pulp defect of another digit has been described. The pedicle is divided after 3 weeks and ROM exercise is then started.

References

1. Moschella F, Cordova A. Reverse homodigital dorsal radial flap of the thumb. Plast Reconstr Surg. 2006;117(3):920–6.
2. Moschella F, Cordova A, Pirrello R, Brunelli F. Anatomic basis for the dorsal radial flap of the thumb: clinical applications. Surg Radiol Anat. 1996;18(3):179–81.
3. Hrabowski M, Kloeters O, Germann G. Reverse homodigital dorsoradial flap for thumb soft tissue reconstruction: surgical technique. J Hand Surg Am. 2010;35(4):659–62.
4. Homann HH, Gojowy D, Sacher M, Schreier D. Homodigitaler Insellappen nach Moschella zur Defektdeckung am Daumen [Moschella island flap for coverage of thumb defects]. Oper Orthop Traumatol. 2020;32(6):494–500. German
5. Qin H, Ma T, Xia J, Zhang W. Comparison of reverse dorsoradial flap for thumb reconstruction: narrow pedicle versus wide pedicle. Arch Orthop Trauma Surg. 2020;140(7):987–92.
6. Bao QY, Xiao CW, Peng F, Han D, Wang T, Gu YD. Restoration of thumb sensibility with innervated reverse homo-digital dorsoradial flap. J Reconstr Microsurg. 2014;30(1):15–20.
7. Sun YC, Chen QZ, Chen J, Gong YP, Gu JH. Reverse dorsoradial flaps for thumb coverage show increased sensory recovery with smaller flap sizes. J Reconstr Microsurg. 2015;31(6):426–33.
8. Sun YC, Gong YP, Chen QZ. A reverse dorsoradial pedicled flap from the thumb for a soft tissue defect in the finger. J Hand Surg Eur. 2015;40(9):1000–1.

Reverse Dorsoulnar or Dorsocubital "Brunelli" Flap

29

Bushra Alhazmi and Abdulaziz Alhujayri

Classification Axial pattern flap, a retrograde homodigital unipedicled skin flap

Vascular Supply [1] Dorsoulnar artery of the thumb.

Innervation [1, 2] Ulnar dorsocollateral nerve (terminal branch of the superficial radial nerve) that can be integrated for a sensate flap

Indications [2]

- Soft tissue loss of palmar aspect of distal thumb.
- Soft tissue loss of the dorsal aspect overlying the proximal or distal phalanx of the thumb (i.e., distal thumb defect with nail avulsion for which microsurgical reconstruction is not an option).
- To cover amputation stump at the level of interphalangeal joint of the thumb.

Contraindications [2]

- Princeps pollicis artery injury.
- Ulnar digital artery injury.
- Significant soft tissue injury affecting the base of the thumb.
- Close proximity of the zone of the injury.

Advantages [1–3]

- Homodigital flap.
- Distally based flap, which can reach the distal areas of the thumb easily.
- Consistent anatomical location of the dorsoulnar artery of the thumb.

B. Alhazmi · A. Alhujayri (✉)
Plastic Surgery Division, Department of Surgery, Ministry of National Guard - Health Affairs, King Abdullah International Medical Research Center, Riyadh, Saudi Arabia

O. Almeshal et al. (eds.), *Soft Tissue Reconstruction of the Hand: Loco-regional and Distant Flaps Selection and Approach*,
https://doi.org/10.1007/978-981-16-9945-0_29

- Providing reasonable texture for dorsal surface reconstruction.
- Minimal donor site morbidity.
- Possible primary closure of the donor site.
- Early postoperative mobility of the thumb.

Disadvantages [2–5]
- Meticulous dissection.
- Overlapping of the pedicle which may require another surgery for debulking of the flap.
- Poor sensory recovery (10 mm 2PD to protective sensation).
- Color mismatch between volar and dorsal skin when attempting volar resurfacing.
- Hair growth on the donor area.

Marking Technique [1, 3, 4]
- A Doppler is used to better delineate the arterial axis of the flap till the pivot point.
- At the level of the neck of the first phalanx, the artery course averages 1 cm from the median axis of the thumb (Fig. 29.1).
- The area of the dorsal arcade of the proximal nail fold is marked, 9 mm proximal to the cuticle.
- The site overlying the palmar anastomosis located in the neck of the first phalanx is marked 2.5 cm proximal to the cuticle.
- According to the defect size, the skin paddle of the flap is marked on the ulnodorsal surface of the MCP joint, centered on the nutrient artery.
- Raising the flap proximal to this area might jeopardize the flap as the dorsoulnar collateral artery travels toward the palmar area and does not supply the remaining dorsal skin of the first intercarpal space.

Surgical Technique [1, 3, 4, 6, 7]
- The procedure is done under general or locoregional anesthesia with tourniquet control.
- The skin paddle is incised, and the flap is elevated in a proximal to distal direction.
- Then, the skin is incised along the marking of the ulnar dorsocollateral artery, being very superficial to avoid injury to the artery underneath.
- Two skin flaps are raised distal to the flap toward the pedicle from the latter incision in a radial and ulnar direction, with special attention not to injure the subcutaneous tissue.
- Isolating the artery during dissection should not be performed as it would easily jeopardize its integrity; instead, a band of subcutaneous tissue measuring approximately 1 cm in width is harvested en bloc centered on the vascular course and leaving the aponeurosis in situ.
- The dissection is performed in a subfascial plane just superficial to the paratenon until the desired pivot point is reached.

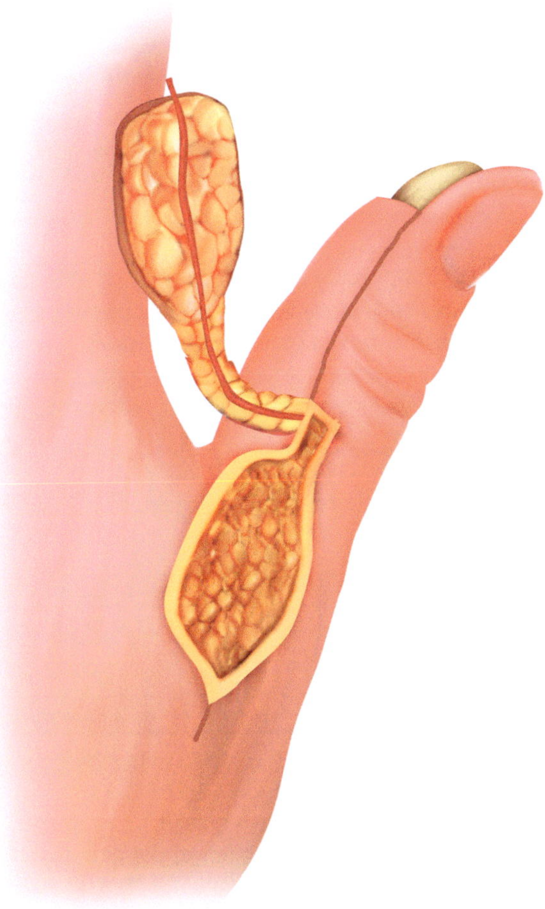

Fig. 29.1 The proposed flap harvest site. The flap is marked on the dorsoulnar side of the thumb. The axis of the flap is centered on the nutrient artery. Dissection is performed in a subfascial plane just superficial to the paratenon till reaching the desired pivot point. A band of subcutaneous tissue is harvested en bloc centered on the vascular course to protect the pedicle. The flap is rotated toward the defect and the donor site is closed primarily based on the width of the flap

- The flap can be pedicled distally at one of two levels:
  - The level of the proximal nail fold arcade (arterial arcade of the nail matrix) (i.e., for volar resurfacing, distal amputation stump coverage, or dorsal resurfacing of the distal area), where dissection should be limited to 1 cm proximal to the nail cuticle.
  - The level of the neck of the first phalanx representing the area of palmar anastomosis (i.e., for more proximal defects), where dissection of the pedicle should be limited to 2.5 cm proximal to the nail cuticle.
- If a sensate flap is intended, the dorsocollateral nerve of the thumb can be harvested after performing the proximal incision.
- The nerve can be located within 1–2 cm from the median axis of the thumb.

- The nerve 2 cm or more from the proximal end of the flap is divided to provide sufficient length for coaptation to one of the palmar digital nerves.
- After the flap is fully mobilized and rotated to the defect area, the tourniquet is released, and flap perfusion is assessed.
- Hemostasis is secured.
- The flap is inset and secured in a tension-free manner.
- The pedicle is secured carefully to avoid subsequent compression.
- A cutaneous tail can be included, which avoids tunneling the pedicle and allows for tension-free closure.
- Terán et al. proposed raising a strip of adipofascial tissue extending from the proximal edge of the flap to facilitate primary closure of the donor site and reduce the risk of first web space contracture.
- Covering the pedicle (and the adipofascial extension if used) with a split-thickness skin graft (STSG) can be done to minimize compression over the pedicle.
- Tension-free closure of the donor site can be done primarily if feasible, with a random local flap (i.e., rotation flap) or with a FTSG.

Postop Care [6]
- Coban tape is applied first week postoperatively for 2–3 months to help decrease the bulkiness of the flap.

Complications [1, 3, 6]
- Distal margin necrosis.
- Vascular compromise (i.e., from compression over the pedicle).
- Flap failure (i.e., when the skin paddle is harvested proximal to the MCP joint, thus excluding the nutrient artery).
- Sensory loss over the dorsum of the thumb and possible neuroma formation in cases where the terminal branch of the radial sensory nerve is harvested.
- Reduced ROM of the MCP joint and first webspace contracture (with moderate-to-large flaps).

Variants
- Cross-finger flap [1, 3, 5]: the flap can be used as a cross-finger flap to reconstruct a pulp defect of another digit [1]. The pedicle is divided at day 15 after performing the clamping test to ensure the independence of the flap (Fig. 29.1) [1].
- Osteocutaneous flap [8, 9]: the first metacarpal receives multiple vascular branches from the proximal continuation of dorsoulnar artery. A vascularized bone from the dorsoulnar aspect of the first metacarpal can be harvested accordingly along with the overlying skin as an alternative option to reconstruct a composite osteocutaneous defect of the distal phalanx.

Case

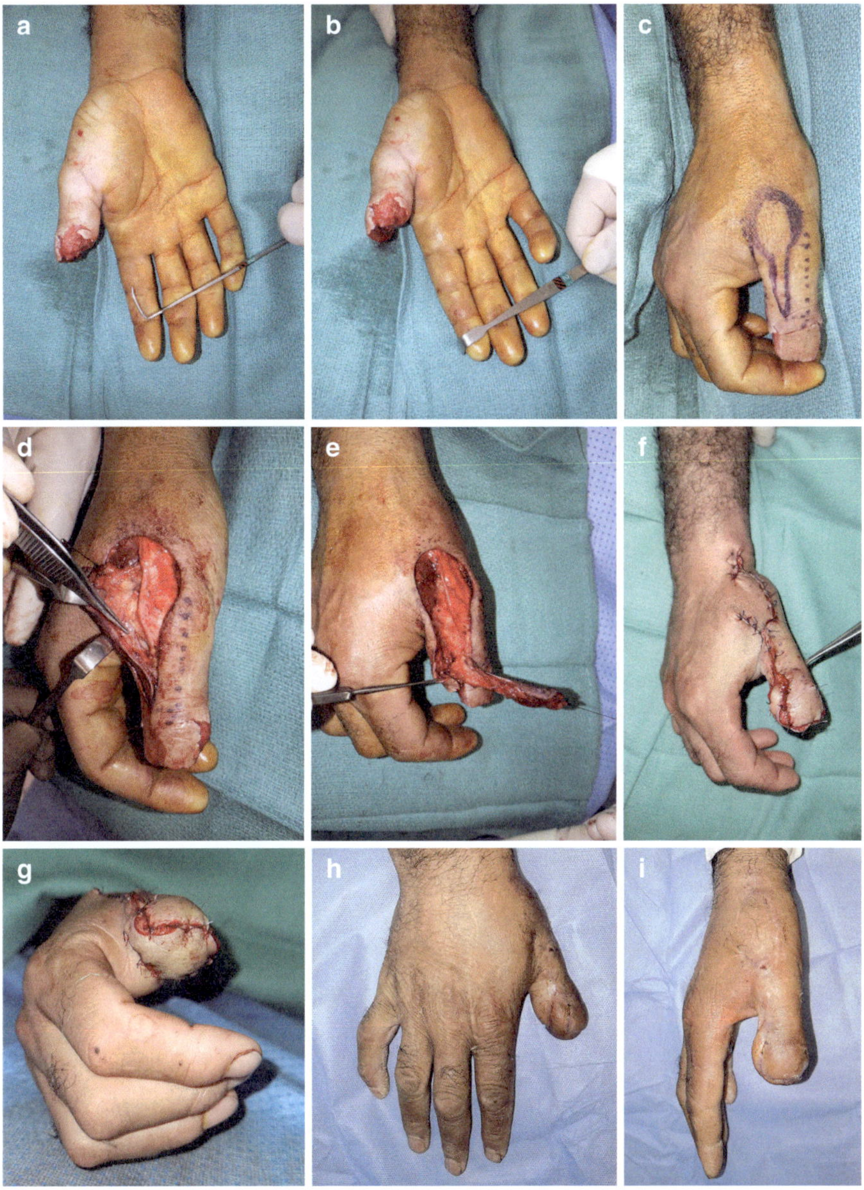

Case 29.1 Intraoperative photos of a patient who presented with traumatic amputation of the distal phalanx of the thumb as seen in (**a**) and (**b**). After good irrigation and washout, coverage was planned with reversed dorsoulnar flap that was marked as shown in (**c**). The flap was then raised based on ulnar dorsocollateral artery as in (**d**). Then, it was rotated to the defect as seen in (**e**). The flap was inset and the donor site was closed with random transposition flap as seen in (**f**) and (**g**). Follow-up assessment at two months is shown in (**h**) and (**i**) with good soft tissue coverage

References

1. Brunelli F, Vigasio A, Valenti P, Gr B. Arterial anatomy and clinical application of the dorsoulnar flap of the thumb. J Hand Surg Am. 1999;24(4):803–11.
2. Slutsky D. Neurosensory pedicled flaps to the hand. Atlas Hand Clin. 2005;10(1):141–70.
3. Adani R, Mugnai R, Petrella G. Reconstruction of traumatic dorsal loss of the thumb: four different surgical approaches. Hand (N Y). 2019;14(2):223–9.
4. Rehim S, Chung K. Local flaps of the hand. Hand Clin. 2014;30(2):137–51.
5. Kumar VP, Satku K, Liu J. The brunelli reversed flow pedicle flap from the thumb. Plast Reconstr Surg. 1996;98(7):1298–301.
6. Terán P, Carnero S, Miranda R, Trillo E, Estefanía M. Refinements in dorsoulnar flap of the thumb: 15 cases. J Hand Surg Am. 2010;35(8):1356–9.
7. Green's operative hand surgery, 6th edition.
8. Pelissier P, Pistre V, Casoli V, Lim A, Martin D, Baudet J. Dorso-ulnar osteocutaneous reverse flow flap of the thumb. J Hand Surg Br. 2001;26(3):207–11.
9. Cavadas PC. Reverse osteocutaneous dorsoulnar thumb flap. Plast Reconstr Surg. 2003;111(1):326–9.

Part V

Pedicled Flaps: Regional Flaps

Adipo-Fascial Flaps

30

Abdullaziz S. Alazzam and Abdulaziz Alhujayri

Classification Random, homodigital

Vascular Supply [1–3] Random blood supply—mainly dorsal branches of the proper digital artery

Innervation Usually, it is not innervated and it depends on the recipient bed for protective sensation. However, there are described variants that include the dorsal sensory branch for coaptation.

Indications [1, 4]
- Coverage of complex dorsal digital wounds as a simple skin graft coverage would not be a valid option because of the exposed bone or tendons.

Contraindications [1]
- Unstable skeletal structure.
- Fingers with compromised vascularity.
- Partial degloving injuries.

Advantages [1, 5, 6]
- Simple, reliable, and easily performed.
- Pliable and thin that can be turned in any direction.
- Minimal donor site morbidity.
- Sparing the proper digital artery.

A. S. Alazzam · A. Alhujayri (✉)
Plastic Surgery Division, Department of Surgery, Ministry of National Guard - Health Affairs, King Abdullah International Medical Research Center, Riyadh, Saudi Arabia

O. Almeshal et al. (eds.), *Soft Tissue Reconstruction of the Hand: Loco-regional and Distant Flaps Selection and Approach*,
https://doi.org/10.1007/978-981-16-9945-0_30

- Useful in multiple finger defects when traditional options such as cross-finger flap or neurovascular island flaps are not possible.
- A smaller amount of skin graft is required, as the epidermal flap can be placed back on the donor site.

Disadvantages [1]
- Thinner dermal flaps can cause desquamation and later depigmentation.
- Improper deepithelization of the epidermal flap can lead to the development of inclusion cysts.
- Skin grafts need to be of moderate thickness.
- Early mobilization is required to prevent stiffness.

Marking Technique [1, 4]
- The size of the defect is measured, and a template is created.
- The flap is marked as per the template with its base proximal to the defect along the longitudinal axis of the injured digit.
- The flap should be marked with a base-to-length ratio of 1:1.5 to 1:3.
- The flap is designed 2 to 4 mm wider than the defect.
- The flap can be based at the site of the dorsal perforator coming at the joint level to ensure better vascularity (Fig. 30.1).

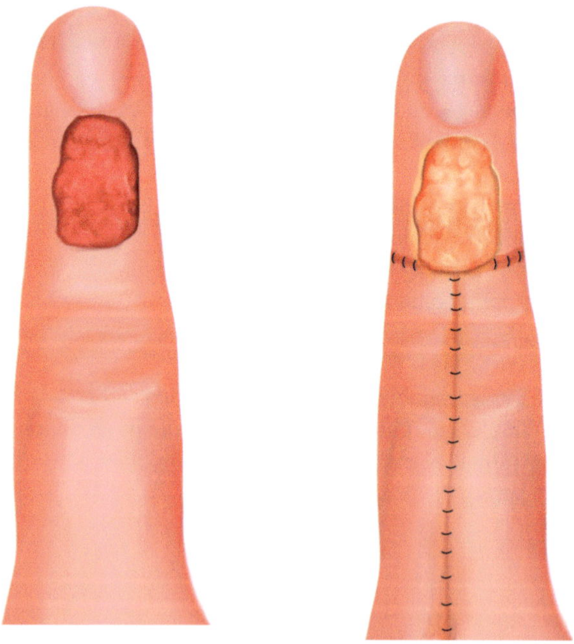

Fig. 30.1 The proposed incision planning of the reverse adipofascial flap. A dorsal longitudinal incision on the digit is done with skin flaps elevated over the dorsal adipofacial tissue. The width of the defect is measured and this is reflected over the area of dissection on the dorsum of the defect with an added 5 mm from the edge of the defect. The flap is then elevated on the dorsum of the digit in a proximal to distal dissection that is stopped 5 mm before the edge of the distal defect. The flap is then flipped toward the defect, and the donor site is closed primarily. The adipofascial flap is then skin grafted

Surgical Technique [1, 4, 7]

- For reverse adipofascial flap, the steps are as follows:
  - The wound is debrided and irrigated properly.
  - K-wire can be used to immobilize the joint in extension.
  - The flap is marked as mentioned above, taking into account the length lost in transposing the flap.
  - Skin is then carefully incised down to the dermal layer and lifted over the underlying adipofascial.
  - The adipofascial flap is dissected distally to proximally from the tendon, making sure to keep the paratenon intact.
  - The dissection of the flap is stopped approximately about 5 mm before the edge of the defect is reached.
  - The adipofascial flap is then turned back on its attached base to cover the defect.
  - A STSG is applied to the raw surface of the turnover flap and any adjacent open areas.
  - The skin over the donor site is sutured over the donor site.

Postop Care [4, 7, 8]

- The first dressing change is done at 3 weeks, at which the K-wire is removed and physiotherapy exercises are started.

Complications [4]

- Flap dehiscence.
- Skin graft loss.
- Stiffness of the adjacent (uninjured) donor finger due to prolonged immobilization.
- Epidermolysis of the skin of the donor site.
- Inclusion cysts.

Variants

- Reverse cross-finger flap [1].
- Braga-Silva turnover adipofascial flaps [6].
- Pedicled adipofascial turnover [9].

Case

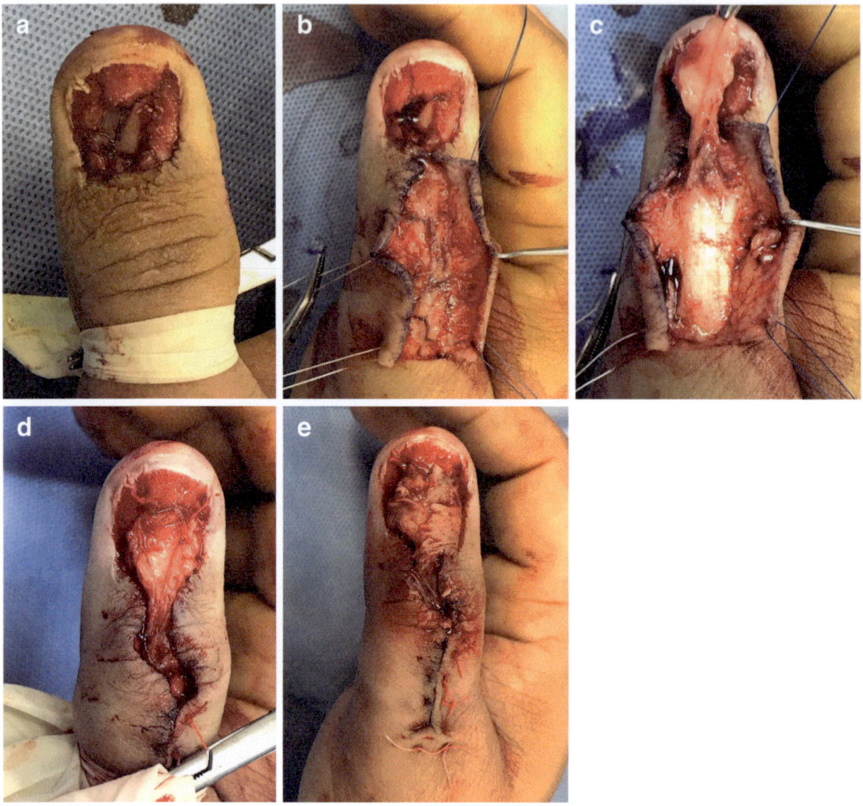

Case 30.1 Intraoperative photo of a patient who presented with a traumatic fingertip injury to the thumb with loss of nail bed and exposed distal phalangeal bone (**a**). After good irrigation and stabilization, coverage of the defect was planned with turnover adipofascial flap and skin graft. The incision was made over the dorsum of the finger to expose the dorsal subcutaneous adipofascial tissue, as seen in (**b**). The adipofascial flap was raised from the proximal to distal direction after assuring good reach with reverse planning and preserving 5 mm of intact tissue before the edge of the defect as in (**c**). The flap was then inset and a skin graft was laid on top of the flap as shown in (**d**) and (**e**)

References

1. Venkatramani H, Varadharajan V. Adipofascial, Transposition, and Rotation Flaps. Hand Clin. 2020;36(1):9–18.
2. Lai CS, Lin SD, Yang CC, Chou CK. The adipofascial turnover flap for complicated dorsal skin defects of the hand and finger. Br J Plast Surg. 1991;44:165–9.
3. Lai CS, Lin SD, Chou CK, Tsai CW. Clinical applications of the adipofascial turn-over flaps for burn wounds. Burns. 1993;19:73–6.
4. Al-Qattan MM. De-epithelialized cross-finger flaps versus adipofascial turnover flaps for the reconstruction of small complex dorsal digital defects: a comparative analysis. J Hand Surg Am. 2005;30(3):549–57.
5. Deal DN, Barnwell J, Li Z. Soft tissue coverage of complex dorsal hand and finger defects using the turnover adipofascial flap. J Reconstr Microsurg. 2011;27(2):133–8.
6. Braga-Silva J, Kuyven CR, Albertoni W, Faloppa F. The adipofascial turn-over flap for coverage of the dorsum of the finger: a modified surgical technique. J Hand Surg Am. 2004;29(6):1038–43.
7. Al-Qattan MM. Technical modifications and extended applications of the distally based adipofascial flap for dorsal digital defects. Ann Plast Surg. 2004;52(2):168–73.
8. Al-Qattan MM. The adipofascial turnover flap for coverage of the exposed distal interphalangeal joint of the fingers and interphalangeal joint of the thumb. J Hand Surg Am. 2001;26(6):1116–9.
9. Voche P, Merle M. The homodigital subcutaneous flap for cover of dorsal finger defects. Br J Plast Surg. 1994;47:435–9.

Finger Propeller Flaps

31

Ali I. Hadadi and Abdulaziz Alhujayri

Classification [1, 2] Adipofasciocutaneous flap.

Vascular Supply [1, 2] Dorsal digital artery perforator.

Innervation [1, 2] Dorsal digital nerve.

Indications [1, 2]
- Small hand defect
- Lack of microsurgical expertise
- The patient not wanting another donor site.

Contraindications [1, 2]
- Large defect
- Defect with greater arc of rotation required
- Donor site within zone of injury
- Crush injury.

Advantages [1–3]
- Technical ease
- Simple and fast in comparison with the free flap
- Lack of microvascular anastomosis
- Minimal donor site morbidity
- Freedom in design and donor site choice
- One-stage procedure.

A. I. Hadadi · A. Alhujayri (✉)
Plastic Surgery Division, Department of Surgery, Ministry of National Guard - Health Affairs, King Abdullah International Medical Research Center, Riyadh, Saudi Arabia

O. Almeshal et al. (eds.), *Soft Tissue Reconstruction of the Hand: Loco-regional and Distant Flaps Selection and Approach*,
https://doi.org/10.1007/978-981-16-9945-0_31

Disadvantages [4]

- Unstable arterial flow
- Pincushion effect
- Limited flap size
- Limited arc of rotation
- Risk of venous congestion.

Marking Technique [1–3]

- The patient is placed in a supine position with the arm abducted on the arm board.
- The marking of the donor site depends on the location of the defect to cover.
- The flap axis is based on the dorsal digital artery perforator on the dorsal ulnar or radial aspect of the finger identified by Doppler signal, which is usually identified at the transverse arch at the joints' level (Fig. 31.1).
- Reverse planning is done to ensure the size and arc of rotation needed.

Surgical Technique [1–3]

- Prepping and draping of the upper limb are conducted under sterile conditions with a tourniquet applied.
- The incision is started under loupe magnification proximally of the designed flap and continues until deep fascia is reached.
- The choice of the dorsal digital artery perforator that is preserved as the vascular pedicle of the flap depends on the following:
  - Course
  - Orientation
  - Pulsatility
  - Accompanying veins number and caliber
  - Caliber
  - Proximity to the edge of the defect.
- After preserving the perforator of choice, an incision of the ulnar and radial aspects of the flap is done.
- Dissection continues proximally to distally superficial to the aponeurosis of extensor tendon with ligation of proximal perforators.
- The pedicle is skeletonized until 2–3 mm of fascia is attached to the perforator to facilitate the arc of rotation.
- The tourniquet is deflated and the adequate blood supply to the flap is confirmed before rotation either clockwise or counterclockwise to cover the defect (choose the smallest angle of rotation and do not exceed 180 degrees).
- The flap is transposed to the recipient site and checked for any twisting or buckling; if any, further dissection is needed.
- The flap capillary refill, color, and bleeding edges are checked; if arterial inflow insufficiency is noted due to vessel spasm, the flap should be put back to the donor site and rinsing with lidocaine or papaverine around the pedicle is performed.

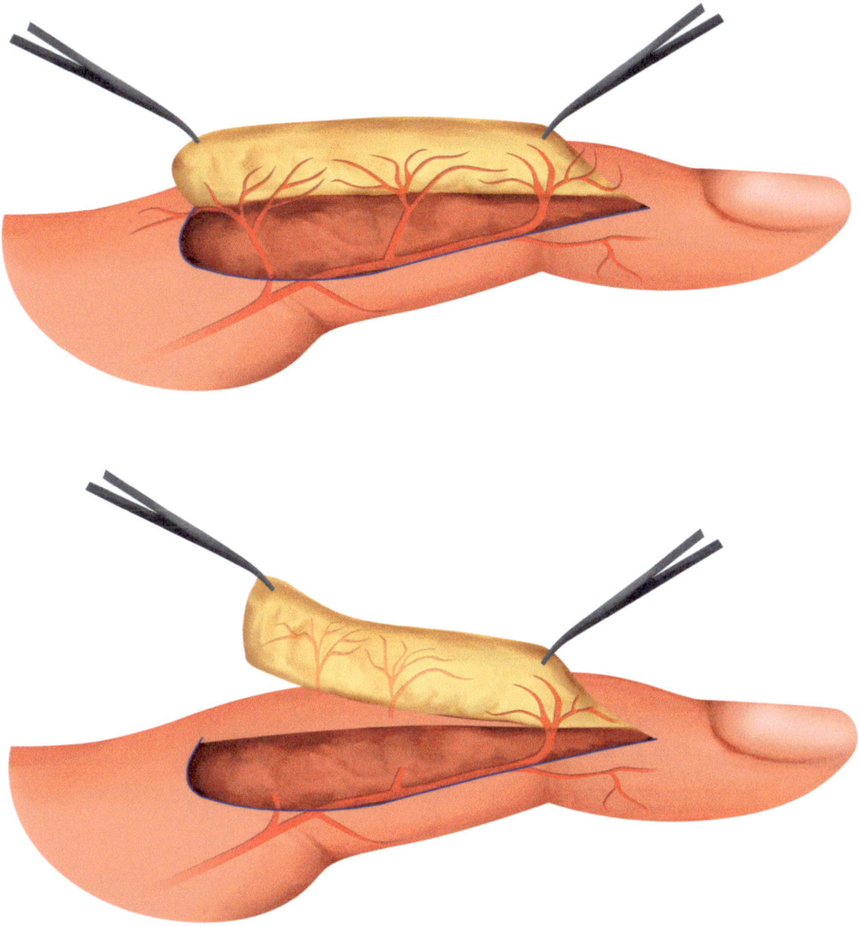

Fig. 31.1 The proposed flap harvest site. The donor site is marked based on the defect to be covered. The flap is marked with its axis based on the dorsal digital artery perforator that is either on the dorsal ulnar or on the radial aspect of the finger. This is usually located at the transverse crease at the joints' level. The flap is then rotated to the defect after skeletonizing the pedicle with an angle of rotation that preferably does not exceed 180 degrees

- If flap arterial inflow insufficiency persisted after derotation and rinsing with lidocaine or papaverine, delay of the flap is recommended.
- The donor site can be closed primarily or covered with a skin graft if needed.

Postop Care [1, 3]

- Splint applied with avoidance of pressure over the flap.
- Ambulation allowed with hand elevation.
- Monitoring the flap for color, temperature, and capillary refill every 2 h in the first days postoperatively.
- Dressing changes as per the surgeon preference.

Complications [3]

- Partial and full flap necrosis
- Arterial insufficiency
- Venous insufficiency.

Variants [5, 6]

- Subcutaneous pedicled propeller flap
- Perforator pedicled propeller flap
- Supercharged propeller flap.

Case

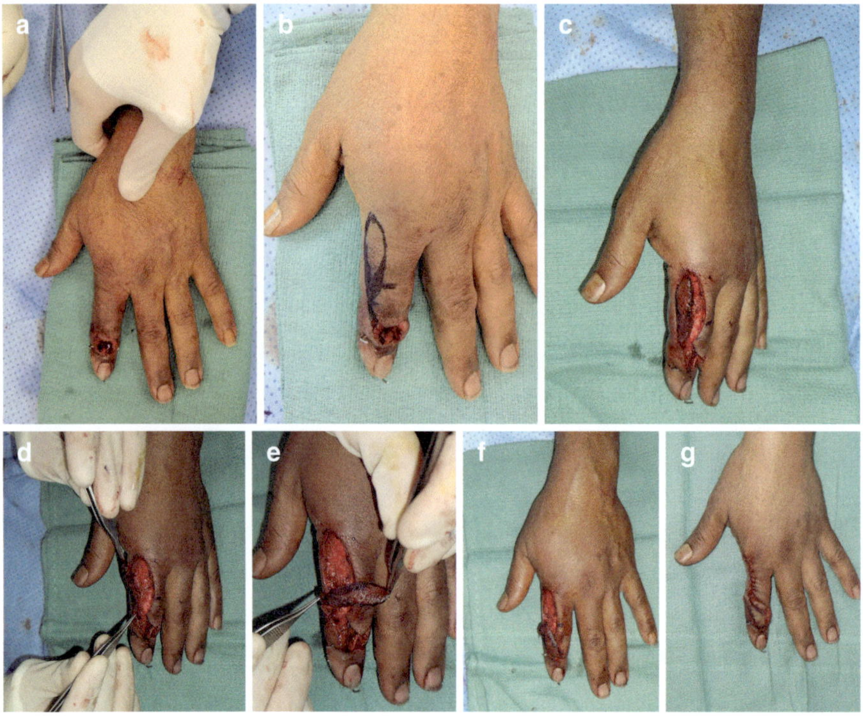

Case 31.1 Intraoperative photo of a patient who presented with index finger distal interphalangeal joint traumatic injury with soft tissue loss as seen in (**a**). After skeletal stabilization with K-wires soft tissue coverage was planned with finger-based propeller flap as marked on the side of the digit based on dorsal radial digital artery perforator after being located with handheld Doppler ultrasound as seen in (**b**). The flap was then raised, making sure to preserve the perforator at the base of the flap as seen in (**c**) and (**d**). The flap was then rotated and propelled at about 160 degrees toward the defect as seen in (**e**). The flap was then inset and the donor site was primary closed, as shown in (**f**) and (**g**)

References

1. Ayestaray B, Ogawa R, Ono S, Hyakusoku H. Propeller flaps: classification and clinical applications. Ann Chir Plast Esthet. 2011;56(2):90–8.
2. Hu H, Chen H, Hong J, et al. Propeller perforator flaps from the dorsal digital artery perforator chain for repairing soft tissue defects of the finger. BMC Surg. 2019;19:188.
3. D'Arpa S, Toia F, Pirrello R, Moschella F, Cordova A. Propeller flaps: a review of indications, technique, and results. BioMed Res Int. 2014.
4. Mitsunaga N, Mihara M, Koshima I, Gonda K, Takuya I, Kato H, Araki J, Yamamoto Y, Yuhei O, Todokoro T, Ishikawa S, Eri U, Mundinger GS. Digital artery perforator (DAP) flaps: modifications for fingertip and finger stump reconstruction. J Plast Reconstr Aesthet Surg. 2010;63(8):1312–7.
5. Pignatti M, Ogawa R, Hallock GG, et al. The "Tokyo" consensus on propeller flaps. Plastic Reconstruct Surg. 2011;127(2):716–22.
6. Blondeel PN, van Landuyt KHI, Monstreyetal SJM. The "Gent" consensus on perforator flap terminology: preliminary definitions. Plastic Reconstruct Surg. 2003;112(5):1378–82.

Dorsal Island Digital (Axial) Flap

32

Abdullaziz S. Alazzam and Nawaf Alohaideb

Classification [1, 2]
- Non-innervated
- Innervated.

Vascular Supply [1–3]
- Dorsal branch of proper digital artery.

Innervation [1, 2]
- Dorsal branch of the digital nerve
- Dorsal digital nerve.

Indications [2]
- Fingertip soft tissue defects
- Finger pulp defects
- Volar aspect of the finger
- Radial aspect of the index finger and the ulnar aspect of the little finger.

Contraindications [1, 6]
- Peripheral arterial disease
- Injuries to the branch, pedicle, or donor site.

Advantages [1, 2, 4–6]
- Simultaneous coverage of multiple finger defect
- Single-stage procedure

A. S. Alazzam · N. Alohaideb (✉)
Plastic Surgery Division, Department of Surgery, Ministry of National Guard - Health Affairs, King Abdullah International Medical Research Center, Riyadh, Saudi Arabia

O. Almeshal et al. (eds.), *Soft Tissue Reconstruction of the Hand: Loco-regional and Distant Flaps Selection and Approach*,
https://doi.org/10.1007/978-981-16-9945-0_32

- Sensory reconstruction in important anatomical regions
- Minimal donor site morbidity
- Brief immobilization
- Sparing other fingers as donor sites.

Disadvantages [1, 2, 4]
- Limited flap size
- Graft contracture
- Extensor tendon adhesion
- Hypersensitivity or symptomatic neuroma.

Marking Technique [1, 2]
- Distal phalanx defects: flap harvest from the dorsum of the middle phalanx (Fig. 32.1).
- Middle and distal phalanx defects: flap harvest from the dorsum of the middle and proximal phalanx.
- The designed flap size 10% to 15% larger than the defect.
- According to the defect location, select the nearest uninjured dorsal branches of the digital artery to the defect as the vascular pedicle of the flap.

Surgical Technique [1–3, 5]
- According to the marking, the initial incision is made along the proximal edges of the flap.
- The two suitable superficial sensory nerve branches distributed to the flap are identified and then cut off at the initial point. (This step is for defects that require restoring sensation, such as pulp of the finger, radial aspect of the index, and ulnar aspect of the little finger.)
- The flap is raised above the extensor tendon with care to keep the paratenon intact.
- Pedicle dissection is made in the volar direction to the pivot point toward the digital artery branching off the dorsal branch.
- For better blood supply for the flap, at least 5 mm wide soft tissue surrounding the artery pedicle also provides better venous drainage.
- The flap is transferred to the recipient site through a subcutaneous tunnel.
- Hemostasis is performed after tourniquet release.
- The subcutaneous tunnel of the vascular pedicle should be as deep as possible to avoid pedicle compression.
- For sensation restoration, a tension-free aponeurorrhaphy with 9–0 nylon suture is performed between the two sensory nerves of the flap and both cut ends of the digital nerves at the recipient wound.
- The flap then is sutured loosely to the defect.
- The donor site is covered with a skin graft and bolstered with the tie-over dressing.

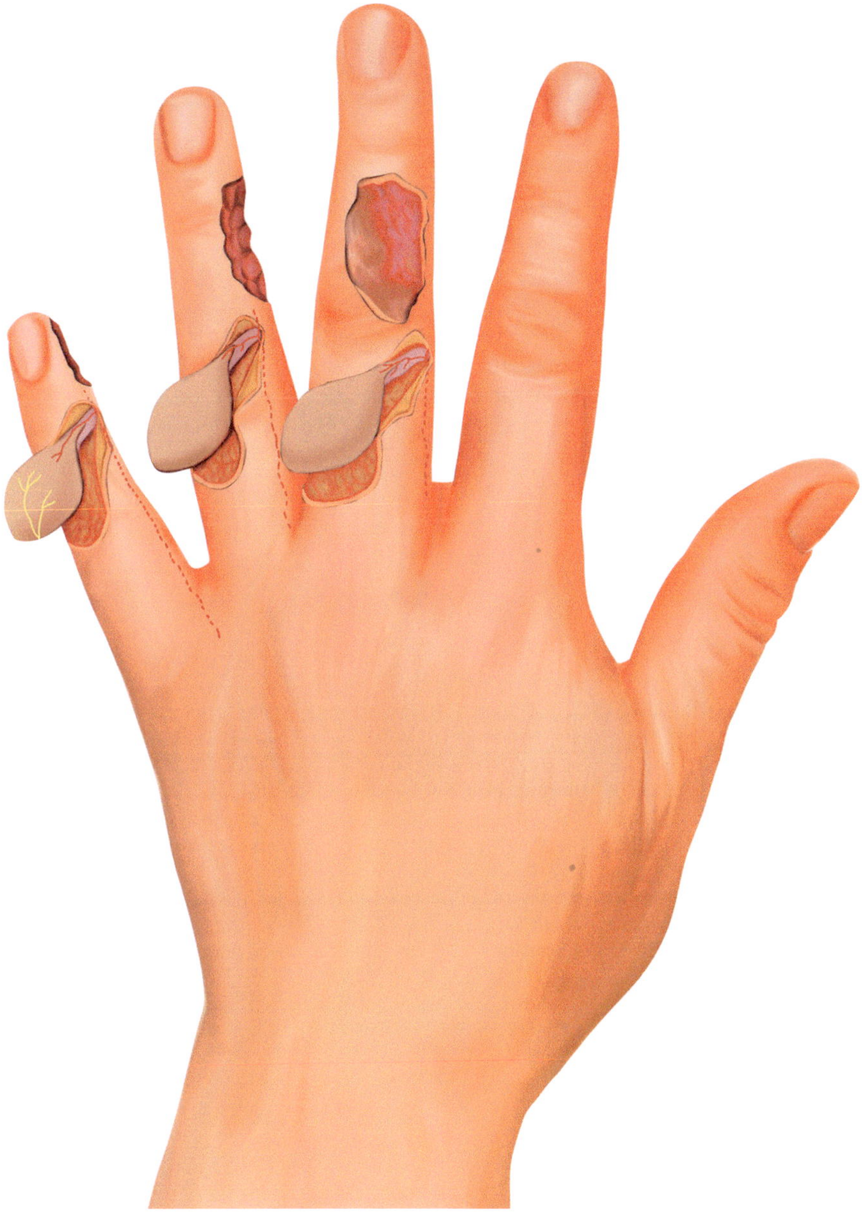

Fig. 32.1 The proposed flap donor site on the dorsum of the middle or the proximal phalanx that is based on the dorsal branch of the proper digital artery as a pedicle. The flap is elevated with a plane over the extensor tendon paratenon. The flap is then rotated to the volar surface defect for coverage and the donor site is skin-grafted

Postop Care [2, 5]

- Hand elevation helps minimize venous congestion.
- For patients who underwent nerve repair, a splint is used for protection, with the interphalangeal joint in full extension and the metacarpophalangeal joint in 70 degrees of flexion.
- The splint is removed at 3 weeks and active ROM exercises are started with the help of a physiotherapist.

Complications [2]

- Flap venous congestion
- Donor site morbidity
- Skin graft contracture
- Hypersensitivity or symptomatic neuroma.

Variants [3, 5, 6]

- Cross-finger flap
- Transposition flap
- Heterodigital reverse-flow neurovascular flap.

References

1. Chen C, Tang P, Zhang L, Li X, Zheng Y. Repair of multiple finger defects using the dorsal homodigital island flaps. Injury. 2013;44(11):1582–8.
2. Chen C, Tang P, Zhang X. The dorsal homodigital island flap based on the dorsal branch of the digital artery: a review of 166 cases. Plast Reconstr Surg. 2014;133(4):519e–29e.
3. Zhang X, Shao X, Zhu M, Jiang R, Feng Y, Ren C. Repair of a palmar soft tissue defect of the proximal interphalangeal joint with a transposition flap from the dorsum of the proximal phalanx. J Hand Surg Eur. 2013;38(4):378–85.
4. Li YF, Cui SS. Innervated reverse island flap based on the end dorsal branch of the digital artery: surgical technique. J Hand Surg Am. 2005;30(6):1305–9.
5. Chen C, Tang P, Zhang X. Sensory reconstruction of a finger pulp defect using a dorsal homodigital island flap. Plast Reconstr Surg. 2012;130(5):1077–86.
6. Yildirim S, Avci G, Akan M, Aköz T. Complications of the reverse homodigital island flap in fingertip reconstruction. Ann Plast Surg. 2002;48(6):586–92.

Reverse Radial Forearm Flap

33

Abdulaziz Alshenaifi and Nawaf Alohaideb

Classification [1] Type B fascial or fasciocutaneous flap.

Vascular Supply [1–6] Retrograde flow from complete palmer arches supplied by ulnar artery and venous drainage through venae comitantes. (The backflow through venae comitantes can be blocked by valve action; however, with increased venous pressure secondary to venous denervation, backflow through venous valves is allowed.)

Innervation [1–3] Lateral antebrachial cutaneous nerve.

Indications [3]
- Reconstruction of soft tissue defects in hand palmar or dorsal surfaces, first web-space, and dorsal thumb.

Contraindications [1, 3]
- Preexisting injuries to the wrist distal forearm area or radial artery.
- Abnormal Allen's test indicative of incomplete arch.

Advantages
- Used for the reconstruction of bones and soft tissue defects
- Innervated flap
- Long pedicle.

A. Alshenaifi · N. Alohaideb (✉)
Plastic Surgery Division, Department of Surgery, Ministry of National Guard - Health Affairs, King Abdullah International Medical Research Center, Riyadh, Saudi Arabia

O. Almeshal et al. (eds.), *Soft Tissue Reconstruction of the Hand: Loco-regional and Distant Flaps Selection and Approach*,
https://doi.org/10.1007/978-981-16-9945-0_33

Disadvantages [3]

- Needing donor site coverage
- Hair-bearing skin
- Possible injury to the superficial radial nerve
- Radial artery proximal ligation
- Venous congestion.

Marking Technique [1–6]

- The patient is placed in a supine position with the arm abducted on the arm table.
- It can be done under general anesthesia or regional anesthesia.
- Prepping and draping should include the whole upper limb and one lower limb for possible skin graft or vein graft harvest.
- A sterile tourniquet is applied.
- Allen's test is performed to confirm the continuity of the deep palmar arch or preoperative angiography; however, the test can be inaccurate.
- The arch's integrity can be examined intraoperatively by making a small incision over the distal radial artery, then applying a microvascular clamp and checking the flow distally; if present, this means that the arch is complete and it is safe to perform the reverse radial forearm flap.
- The flap can include the volar forearm skin with borders as follows:
  - Ulnar: flexor carpi ulnaris
  - Radial: extensor carpi radialis longus
  - Proximal: antecubital crease
  - Distal: wrist crease
  - Flap axis: Midpoint at antecubital fossa to slightly radial to flexor carpi radialis tendon at wrist crease.
- The distance from the radial styloid (pivot point) to the proximal margin of the dorsal or palmar hand defect is measured and this distance transposed proximally up the anterior surface of the forearm to estimate the size needed for the flap (Fig. 33.1).
- The flap is centralized slightly ulnarly to the radial artery to include thinner and less hair-bearing skin.
- A thin skin paddle can be marked along the radial artery course to prevent skin grafting over the pedicle or skin bridges later.
- If the defect is located more distally, the flap can be designed more proximally over the junction between the proximal and middle thirds of the forearm.

Surgical Technique [1–6]

- The tourniquet with no exsanguination is inflated.
- The proximal ulnar side of the flap is incised and dissected down to fascia with no flap undermining.
- The fascia is incised; then, subfascial dissection is done toward the radial artery.

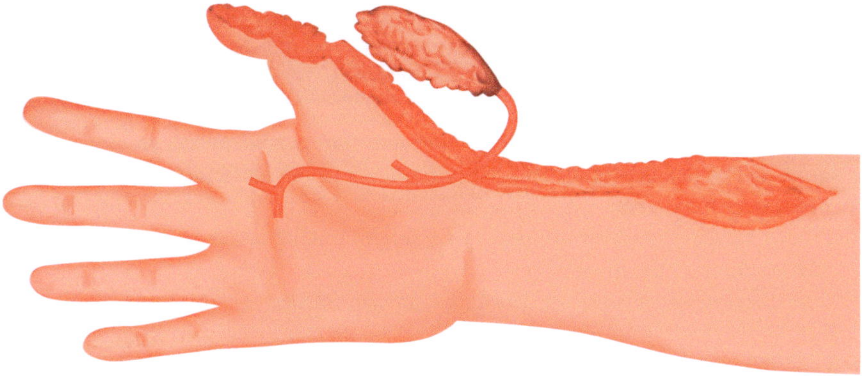

Fig. 33.1 The axis of the flap over the course of the radial artery. The distance from the radial styloid (pivot point) to the proximal margin of the hand defect is measured and this distance is transposed proximally over the anterior surface of the forearm to estimate the size needed for the flap. After flap elevation, the radial artery is ligated proximally and the flap is transposed to the defect

- The medial antebrachial cutaneous nerve and lateral antebrachial cutaneous nerve are identified, which can be included in the flap for sensation.
- The palmaris longus is identified, which also can be harvested as vascularized tendon graft or excluded.
- The paratenon is kept for all tendons.
- Once the dissection reached the intermuscular septum between flexor carpi radialis tendon and brachioradialis, a deep fascial incision over the medial aspect of flexor carpi radialis muscle is made.
- The radial skin incision is made in the same fashion and dissection toward the radial artery is attempted, making sure not to injure the sensory branch of the radial nerve.
- The fascia that is located superficial to the radial artery should be left undisturbed as it contains the septocutaneous perforators that supply the skin flap.
- Deep fascia is sutured to the skin to avoid shearing forces.
- The radial artery is dissected on both sides of the septum and the artery at the pivot point is identified.
- A proximal forearm incision is done for artery ligation and harvest of sensory nerves as needed.
- Dissection deep into the artery is done after the artery is clamped and cut proximally.
- The tourniquet is deflated after clamping the artery proximally and before cutting it to ensure adequate thumb perfusion.

- Proximal to distal dissection is made until reaching the pivot point, not exceeding the radial styloid. The flap is then rotated to the defect, ensuring that the pedicle is not twisted, kinked, or compressed.
- Nerve neurorrhaphy is done if desired.
- In case of any venous congestion after the flap is transposed, leeches can be applied or the superficial vein from the flap can be anastomosed to one of the veins near the defect.
- Arc or rotation can be increased by freeing the radial artery at the snuffbox and can reach up to the thumb tip.
- The donor site can be closed primarily or with STSG.

Postop Care
- Wrist immobilization with slight extension
- Hand elevation on one pillow
- Anticoagulation not routinely needed
- Initiation of physical therapy and scar management after complete flap healing.

Complications
- Possible need for a skin graft
- Skin graft failure over tendons
- Possible cold intolerance
- Flap edema due to interrupted venous drainage
- Hair-bearing flap.

Variants
- Axial pedicled/free radial forearm flap.
- Fascial radial forearm flap.
- Perforator-based radial forearm flap.
- Fasciosteocutanous radial forearm flap.

Case

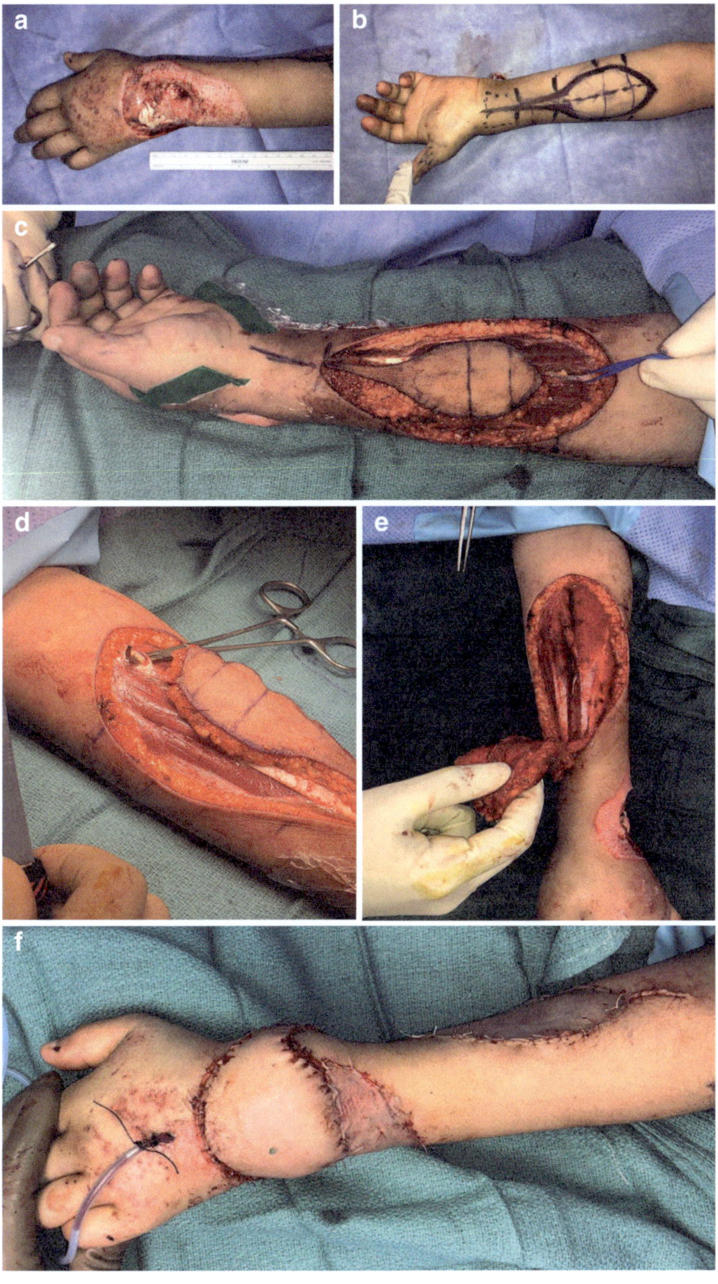

Case 33.1 Intraoperative photo of a patient who presented with dorsal hand and wrist soft tissue defect with exposed bones as shown in (**a**). Coverage was planned with revered radial forearm pedicled flap after ensuring good wound irrigation and washout. Flap marking was done with a template of the defect, ensuring good flap reach with reverse planning as seen in (**b**). The flap was raised from both the radial and ulnar sides with the inclusion of the radial artery, as shown in (**c**) and (**d**). The flap was then transposed to cover the defect with a skin graft applied to the donor area as seen in (**e**) and (**f**)

References

1. Jones NF, Jarrahy R, Kaufman MR. Pedicled and free radial forearm flaps for reconstruction of the elbow, wrist, and hand. Plast Reconstr Surg. 2008;121(3):887–98.
2. Yajima H, Kobata Y, Kawamura K, Shigematsu K, Kawate K, Tamai S. Radial forearm flaps for reconstruction in hand surgery. Scand J Plast Reconstr Surg Hand Surg. 2004;38(2):112–7.
3. Slutsky DJ. Pedicled radial forearm flap. In: The art of microsurgical hand reconstruction. New York, NY: Thieme; 2013. p. 24–32.
4. Akdag O, Karamese M, NebilSelimoglu M, Akatekin A, Abacı M, Sutcu M, Tosun Z. Reverse adipofascial radial forearm flap surgery for soft tissue reconstruction of hand defects. Eplasty. 2016;16:e35.
5. El-Khatib HA, Hammouda AH. Reverse osseofasciocutaneous radial forearm flap for thumb reconstruction: a flap design and case series. J Hand Surg. 2005;30(6):1298–304.
6. Zambacos GJ, Mandrekas AD. The reverse radial forearm flap in reconstruction of the hand. Plastic Reconstruct Surg. 2008;122(6):1979–80. author reply 1980

Radial Artery Perforator Flap

34

Abdulaziz Alshenaifi and Nawaf Alohaideb

Classification [1] Type B fascial or fasciocutaneous flap.

Vascular Supply [1, 3, 5]
- Perforating vessels from radial artery, mainly distal perforators located 1.5 cm proximal to radial styloid.
- Venous drainage through perforator venae comitantes.
- Controversial opinions regarding cephalic vein drainage of the flap.

Innervation Lateral antebrachial cutaneous nerve.

Indications [4]
- Reconstruction of soft tissue defects in hand palmar or dorsal surfaces not distal to metacarpophalangeal joints.

Contraindications [4]
- Preexisting injuries to the wrist distal forearm area or radial artery
- Smoking, venous insufficiency, and diabetes.

Advantages [2]
- Preservation of radial artery
- Reliable blood supply
- Used as an innervated flap.

A. Alshenaifi · N. Alohaideb (✉)
Plastic Surgery Division, Department of Surgery, Ministry of National Guard - Health Affairs, King Abdullah International Medical Research Center, Riyadh, Saudi Arabia

O. Almeshal et al. (eds.), *Soft Tissue Reconstruction of the Hand: Loco-regional and Distant Flaps Selection and Approach*,
https://doi.org/10.1007/978-981-16-9945-0_34

Disadvantages [4, 7]

- Possible need for skin graft
- The maximum size of the flap being smaller and the reach more proximal than that of the traditional axial flap
- Venous congestion.

Marking Technique [1–7]

- The patient is placed in a supine position with the arm abducted on the arm table.
- It can be done under general anesthesia or regional anesthesia.
- Prepping and draping should include the whole upper limb and one lower limb for a possible skin graft.
- A sterile tourniquet is applied.
- Defect size is measured and the distance estimated between pivot point (2–4 cm proximal to radial styloid) and defect.
- The flap is centralized over the radial artery.
- The flap axis is from the midpoint at the antecubital fossa to the radial artery at the wrist crease (Fig. 34.1).
- A thin skin paddle can be marked along the course of RA to prevent skin grafting over the pedicle or skin bridges later.
- The preliminary proximal edge of the flap is drawn and can be adjusted based on the selected perforator and distance from the defect.

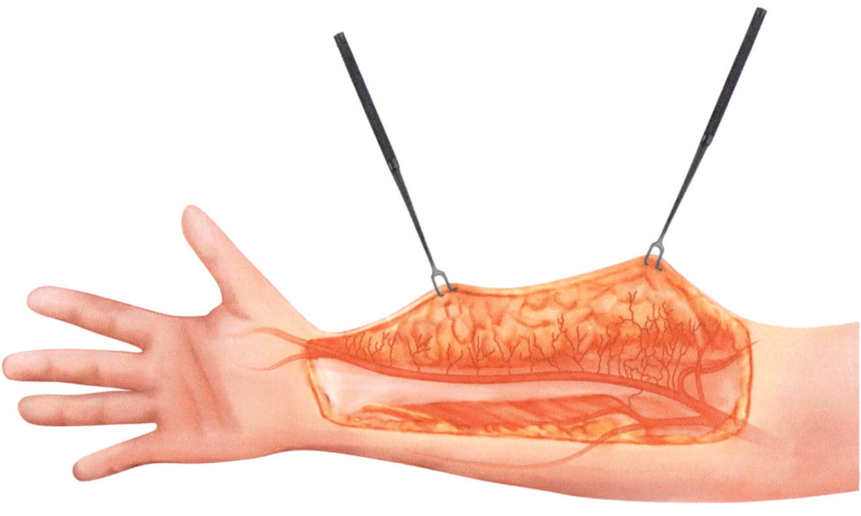

Fig. 34.1 The axis of the flap over the course of the radial artery. Careful dissection is made to ensure that the flap is based on one of the radial artery perforators. The flap is usually raised through subfascial dissection that is advanced toward the radial artery keeping all perforators of interest intact. This is especially true for those 2–4 cm proximal to radial styloid to ensure good flap perfusion in a reverse fashion with intact radial artery proper

Surgical Technique

- The tourniquet with no exsanguination is inflated.
- One side of the flap is incised and dissected down to the fascia with no flap undermining.
- The skin is incised from the wrist crease and connected with a flap incision.
- The fascia is incised and then, subfascial dissection is made toward the radial artery carefully to keep all perforators, especially the ones 2–4 cm proximal to radial styloid.
- The lateral antebrachial cutaneous nerve is preserved, which can be included in the flap for sensation.
- The other side of the flap is incised and the same previous steps are repeated.
- PL is identified, which also can be harvested as vascularized tendon graft or excluded.
- Paratenon is kept for all tendons.
- The sensory branch of the radial nerve is protected.
- Once dissection reaches the septum between BR and FCR, the best perforator is selected based on size (preferably >0.5 mm) and pulsation.
- Deep fascia is sutured to the skin to avoid shearing forces.
- After selection of the desired perforator within the 2–4 cm pivot point, the other proximal ones are ligated while elevating the flap from proximal to distal.
- The proximal edge of the flap is confirmed before starting based on the distance from the pivot point to the proximal edge and defect.
- The tourniquet is deflated and good flap perfusion, adequate perforator pulsation, and Doppler signals are ensured.
- The flap is rotated to the defect and inset.
- The donor site can be closed primarily or with STSG.

Postop Care

- Wrist immobilization with slight extension
- Hand elevation on one pillow
- Anticoagulation not routinely needed
- Initiation of physical therapy and scar management after complete flap healing.

Complications

- Single perforator flap
- Possible need for skin graft.

Variants

- Axial pedicled/free radial forearm flap
- Fascial radial forearm flap
- Perforator-based radial forearm flap
- Osteocutaneous radial forearm flap.

Case

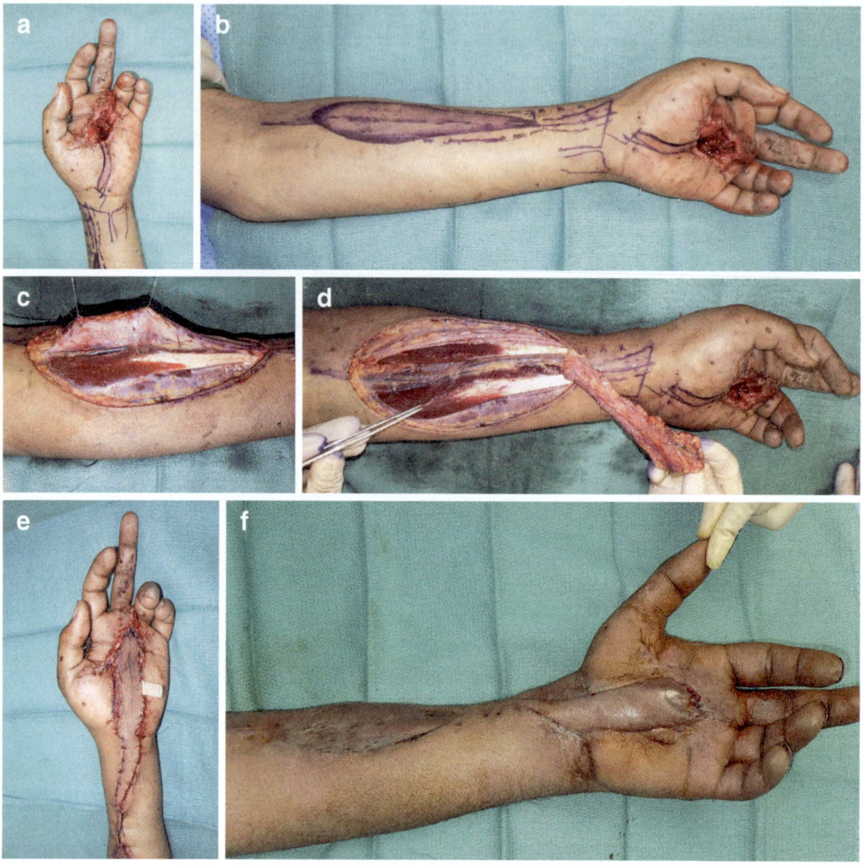

Case 34.1 Intraoperative photo of a patient who had a through-and-through mid-palm gunshot wound (**a**). After good wound irrigation and washout, volar hand defect coverage was planned with a radial artery perforator-based flap. The flap was marked as shown in (**b**). starting with distal radioulnar joint marking then by locating the perforator with handheld Doppler ultrasound. The flap was raised, persevering the perforator at the base of the flap as a reversed fashion flap with intact radial artery continuity as seen in (**c**) and (**d**). The flap was then rotated and was inset to the defect as seen in (**e**). On a subsequent follow-up at six weeks postop, intact soft tissue coverage was ensured as seen in (**f**)

References

1. Chang SM. The distally based radial forearm fascia flap. Plast Reconstr Surg. 1990;85(1):150–1.
2. Hou C, Chang S, Lin J, Song D. Surgical Atlas of perforator flaps a microsurgical dissection technique. Dordrecht: Springer; 2015.
3. Sham E, Masia J, Reddy T. Vascular analysis of radial artery perforator flaps. Ann Maxillofacial Surg. 2018;8(1):66.
4. Ho AM, Chang J. Radial artery perforator flap. J Hand Surg. 2010;35(2):308–11.
5. Saint-Cyr M, Mujadzic M, Wong C, Hatef D, Lajoie AS, Rohrich RJ. The radial artery pedicle perforator flap: vascular analysis and clinical implications. Plastic Reconstruct Surg. 2010;125(5):1469–78.
6. Yamakawa S, Hayashida K. Dorsal hand reconstruction with radial artery perforator-based adipofascial flap. Plast Aesthet Res. 2020;7:24.
7. Matei I, Georgescu A, Chiroiu B, Capota I, Ardelean F. Harvesting of forearm perforator flaps based on intraoperative vascular exploration: clinical experiences and literature review. Microsurgery. 2008;28:321–30.

Fillet Flap (Amputation Cases) 35

Anas M. Alyamani and Feras Alshomer

Classification [1] Regional flap.

Vascular Supply [1]
- Axial pattern flap, type A supplied by digital arteries.

Innervation [2–4]
- Innervation of the flap depends on the presence of sensory nerve within the flap.
- Type A is innervated by digital nerves.

Indications [2]
- Fillet flaps are harvested from a vascularized digit or limb which is partly damaged.
- They are harvested from amputated, discarded, or nonfunctioning or non-salvageable parts.
- Sometimes, normal limbs are used as fillet flaps to reconstruct a defect.

Contraindications [5]
- Absolute contraindications
- Tumor extension in oncological cases
- Relative contraindications
- Infection.

A. M. Alyamani
Plastic Surgery Division, Department of Surgery, Ministry of National Guard - Health Affairs, King Abdullah International Medical Research Center, Riyadh, Saudi Arabia

F. Alshomer (✉)
Division of Plastic Surgery, Department of Surgery, King Abdulaziz Medical City, Ministry of National Guard - Health Affairs. King Abdullah International Medical Research Center, Riyadh, Saudi Arabia

O. Almeshal et al. (eds.), *Soft Tissue Reconstruction of the Hand: Loco-regional and Distant Flaps Selection and Approach*,
https://doi.org/10.1007/978-981-16-9945-0_35

Advantages [3]

- Sensate flap if the nerve is preserved
- Durable coverage
- Excellent color match of the skin.

Disadvantages

- The damaged finger may have precarious vascularity and using the filleted flap from this finger to cover a defect may not be reliable.

Marking Technique

- Flap is designed depending on the defect size and location, ensuring the inclusion of the digital artery within the flap design.
- A palmar incision is designed to utilize the remainder of the dorsal skin flap for coverage (Fig. 35.1).

Surgical Technique [5]

- A longitudinal incision is made. Distally, a circumferential incision is made around the finger at a point 5 mm proximal to the nail fold.
- At the proximal end of the longitudinal incision, it depends on whether the metacarpal of the digit is to be resected or not. If the metacarpal is not to be excised, a transverse incision is made over the dorsum of the finger to create a hinge along the side of the finger opposite the incision. If the metacarpal is excised, the incision is extended proximally.
- The underlying bone and tendons are removed.
- The flap can now be opened and folded onto the primary defect.

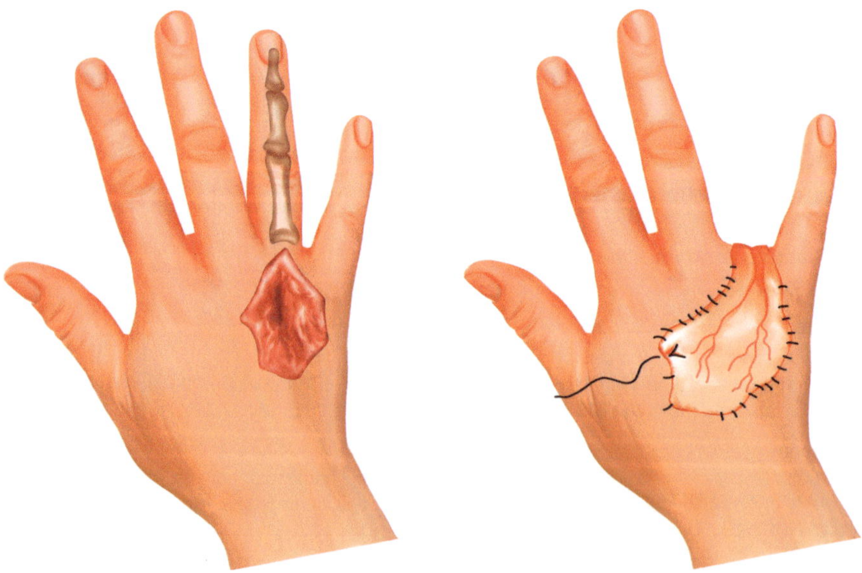

Fig. 35.1 The utility of finger fillet flap in the coverage of hand soft tissue defects. The intact skin of the injured digit is used that is based on intact digital neurovascular bundles in which the bones were amputated and the intact skin cover was transposed to cover the defect

Postop Care

- The flap should be monitored clinically for any sign of congestion, necrosis, or infection.

Complications [1]

- Total or partial flap necrosis
- Hematoma
- Infection.

Variants [2]

- The three types of fillet flaps are as follows: Type A, finger and toe flaps; type B, limb flaps, type C, flaps from intact body parts.
- Flaps can be transferred as pedicled (subclassification 1), island (subclassification 2), and free flap (subclassification 3).

Case

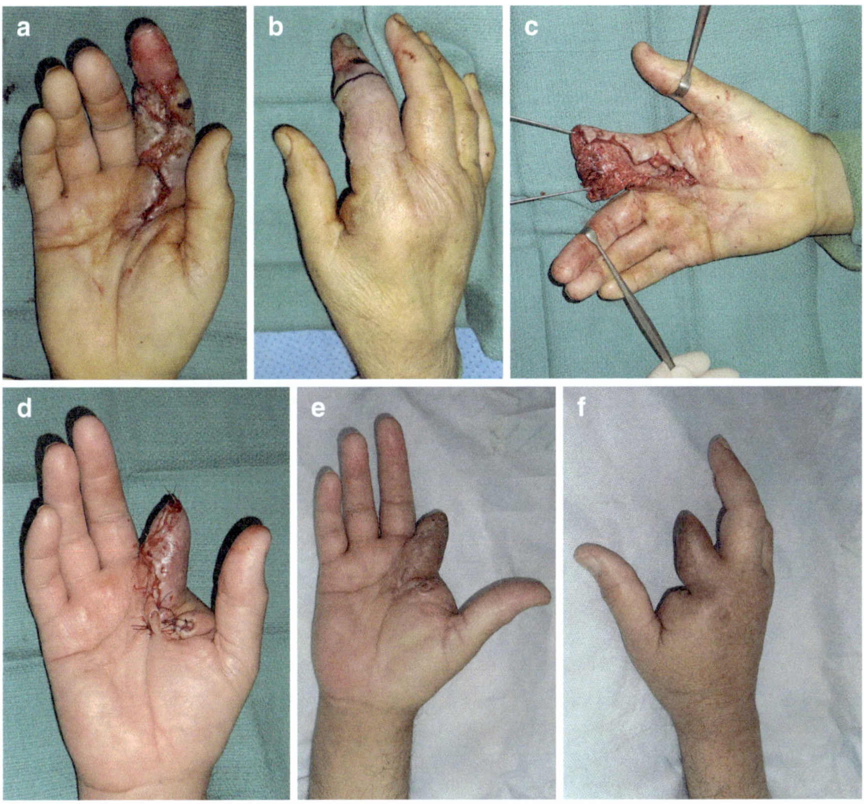

Case 35.1 Intraoperative photo of a patient who had an advanced case of hand flexor tenosynovitis in which there was no response to previous attempts of irrigation and debridement with extensive osteomyelitis (**a**). The patient was taken for index finger amputation with preservation of healthy skin for coverage as fillet flap as marked in (**b**). After removing the bone and infected tissue, healthy skin tissue was preserved, as seen in (**c**). The skin was approximated as seen in (**d**). One-month follow-up is seen in (**e**) and (**f**)

References

1. Küntscher MV, et al. The concept of fillet flaps: classification, indications, and analysis of their clinical value. Plastic Reconstruct Surg. 2001;108(4):885–96.
2. Levin LS, Erdmann D, Germann G. The use of fillet flaps in upper extremity reconstruction. J Am Soc Surg Hand. 2002;2(1):39–44.
3. Schonauer F, Schaden D, Teo TC. Fillet of finger flap for hand resurfacing after tumour excision. Eur J Surg Oncol. 1999;25(4):424–6.
4. Koegel AM, et al. Sensibility of finger fillet flaps on late follow-up evaluation. J Hand Surg. 1995;20(4):679–82.
5. Ayyala HS, et al. The forearm fillet flap:'spare parts' reconstruction for forequarter amputations. Case Reports Plast Surg Hand Surg. 2019;6(1):95–98.

36 Reverse Posterior Interosseous Artery Flap

Nawaf Alohaideb

Classification [1] Fasciocutaneous flap.

Vascular Supply Posterior interosseous artery.

Innervation N/A.

Indications [1–4]
- It can be used to cover the thumb up to the interphalangeal joint, first webspace, proximal palm, anterior wrist, and dorsal hand defects up to the level of metacarpophalangeal joints.

Contraindications [5]
- Injuries to the distal forearm and wrist areas.

Advantages [5]
- Sparing main forearm vessels
- Thin flap
- Sufficient arc of rotation
- Possible for vascularized bone graft harvest with the flap.

Disadvantages [5]
- Absence anastomosis distally in 5% of people
- Not sensate
- Possible injury to deep branch of radial nerve
- Visually exposed donor site of the flap.

N. Alohaideb (✉)
Plastic Surgery Division, Department of Surgery, Ministry of National Guard - Health Affairs, King Abdullah International Medical Research Center, Riyadh, Saudi Arabia

O. Almeshal et al. (eds.), *Soft Tissue Reconstruction of the Hand: Loco-regional and Distant Flaps Selection and Approach*,
https://doi.org/10.1007/978-981-16-9945-0_36

Marking Technique [1, 5–8]

- Doppler sonography is advisable before confirming the presence of anastomosis distally between the anterior and posterior interosseous arteries.
- The patient is placed in a supine position with the arm abducted on the arm table.
- It can be done under general anesthesia or regional anesthesia using a partially exsanguinated tourniquet to keep venae comitantes filled with blood for better visibility.
- The course of the posterior interosseous artery is marked by drawing a line connecting the lateral epicondyle of the humerus to the center of the dorsal radioulnar joint. Along the course of the artery, there are 7–14 cutaneous perforators supplying the skin and the fascia.
- The flap should be centered over the middle third or about 9 cm from the lateral epicondyle with a maximum size of 12 × 8 cm along the drawn line (Fig. 36.1).
- The rotation point of the flap is 2–3 cm from the center of the distal radioulnar joint.
- Most of the important perforators are located over the distal to the midline of the axis.

Surgical Technique [1–10]

- The first step is to make a small incision over the distal edge of the marked flap to identify and confirm the presence of anastomosis between anterior and posterior interosseous arteries.
- Once anastomosis is confirmed, the ulnar border is incised and dissection starts over the proximal two-thirds of the flap as the pedicle of the posterior interosse-

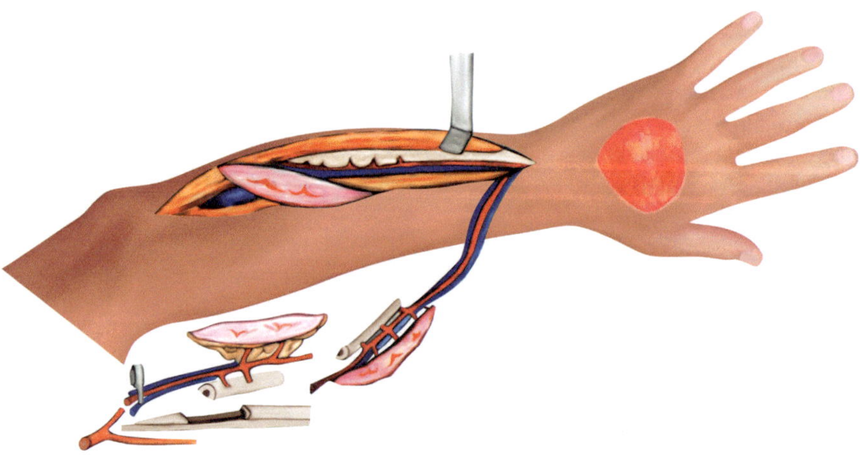

Fig. 36.1 The course of the posterior interosseous artery is marked by drawing a line connecting the lateral epicondyle of the humerus to the center of the dorsal radioulnar joint. The flap should be centered over the middle third of the marked line. The rotation point of the flap is 2–3 cm from the center of the distal radioulnar joint. Different variations of the flap are also shown as an osteofasciocutaneous flap

ous artery is bigger and easier to find and also the muscle belly of extensor carpi ulnaris is easily identified at this level.
- Fascia over extensor carpi ulnaris is incised and dissection is carried out until reaching the septum; the intermuscular septum is exposed by retracting the extensor carpi ulnaris muscle ulnarly.
- The separation between the artery and nerve is done carefully, making sure not to injure any muscular branches of the nerve lying radial to and deep into the artery.
- The radial border of the marked flap is incised and dissection is carried out on a subfascial plane until reaching the intermuscular septum between extensor digiti minimi and extensor carpi ulnaris.
- Once the septum is identified, septal perforators are preserved and muscular perforators are ligated.
- The posterior interosseous artery is followed proximally and clamped once reaching the distal border of the supinator muscle.
- The tourniquet is released and perfusion to the flap is checked before the separation of the pedicle.
- Hemostasis is achieved; then, separation of the septum is done proximally to distally until reaching the anastomosis point (pivot point of the flap).
- Transposition of the flap to the defect is done by either creating a subcutaneous tunnel or incising the skin toward the defect.
- The donor site of the flap is closed primarily if the width of the flap permits or using a STSG to cover the defect.

Postop Care [4, 5, 8]
- The wrist is immobilized in 20° extension and the metacarpophalangeal joint is flexed 70° for 2 weeks in a short arm splint.
- The limb is kept elevated over a pillow.
- The flap should be monitored regularly to check vascularity.
- Intravenous antibiotics are continued for 5 days.
- Physiotherapy and scar management are started once the immobilization period is completed and the flap is healed with its donor area.

Complications [11]
- Partial flap necrosis
- Complete flap necrosis
- Donor site graft loss
- Venous congestion
- Infection
- Absence of anastomosis between anterior and posterior interosseous artery distally.

Variants
- Posterior interosseous sensate flap
- Posterior interosseous fascial flap
- Posterior interosseous osteo-fascio-cutaneous flap
- Posterior interosseous flap with vascularized tendon or muscle.

Case

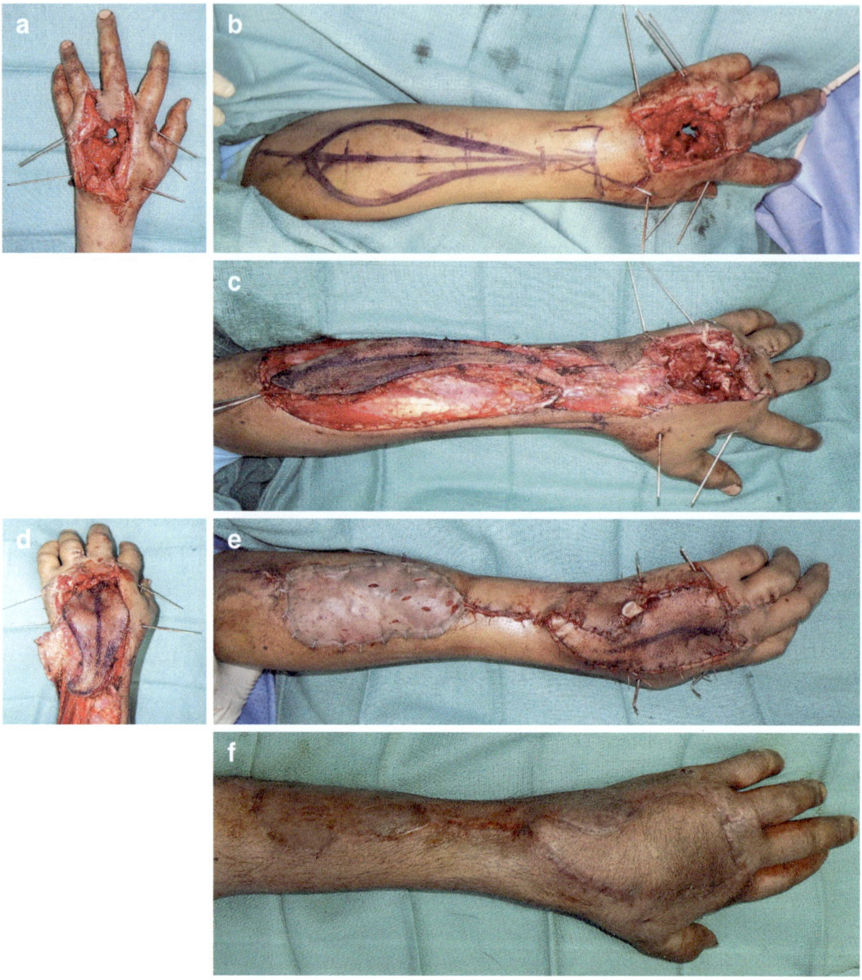

Case 36.1 Intraoperative photo of a patient who presented with a traumatic gunshot wound to the hand with through-and-through in the mid-palmar area with soft tissue and bone loss as seen in (**a**). After wound irrigation and skeletal stabilization with K-wires, coverage of dorsal hand defect was planned with a reverse PIA flap. The flap was marked over the dorsum of the forearm along the course between lateral epicondyle of the humerus to the dorsal radioulnar joint ending about 2–3 cm from the dorsal radioulnar joint as a pivot point as seen in (**b**). Flap was then raised, preserving the septum between extensor digiti minimi and extensor carpi ulnaris with adipofascial paddle that the communicating vessel as in (**c**). The flap was then transposed to the defect as in (**d**). The flap was then inset and the donor site was skin-grafted as seen in (**e**). Follow-up assessment at 3 months after flap coverage is seen in (**f**)

References

1. Chao JD, Huang JM, Wiedrich TA. Local hand flaps. J Am Soc Surg Hand. 2001;1(1):25–44.
2. Zenn M, Jones G. Reconstructive surgery: anatomy, technique, and clinical application. 2012.
3. Eo SR, Hwang SH, Hong KY, Lim SA, Lee GJ. Revisiting the posterior interosseous artery flap. Arch Hand Microsurg. 2018;23(3):195.
4. El-Sabbagh A, Zeina A, El-Hadidy A-M, El-Din A. Reversed posterior interosseous flap: safe and easy method for hand reconstruction. J Hand Microsurg. 2016;03(02):66–72.
5. Hierner R, Putz R, Bishop AT, Shen Z, Wilhelm K. Flaps in hand and upper limb reconstruction: surgical anatomy, operative techniques, and differential therapy. 2014.
6. Krishnan KG. An illustrated handbook of flap-raising techniques. Stuttgart: Thieme; 2008.
7. Acharya AM, Bhat AK, Bhaskaranand K. The reverse posterior interosseous artery flap: technical considerations in raising an easier and more reliable flap. J Hand Surg. 2012;37(3):575–82.
8. Khurram MF, Maurya SK, Yaseen M, Chowdhry M. Reverse posterior interosseous artery flap: a reliable, comfortable and versatile flap for coverage of soft tissue defects of hand. J Wound Manage Res. 2020;16(2):73–9.
9. Zancolli E, Angrigiani C. Posterior interosseous island forearm flap. J Hand Surg. 1988;13(2):130–5.
10. Balakrishnan G, Sampath Kumar B, Hussain SA. Reverse-flow posterior interosseous artery flap revisited. Plastic Reconstruct Surg. 2003;111(7):2364–9.
11. Puri V, Mahendru S, Rana R. Posterior interosseous artery flap, fasciosubcutaneous pedicle technique: a study of 25 cases. J Plastic Reconstruct Aesthetic Surg. 2007;60(12):1331–7.

Dorsal Ulnar Artery Flap

37

Nawaf Alohaideb

Classification [1] Fasciocutaneous flap

Vascular Supply Dorsal branch of the ulnar artery (ulnar cubitodorsal artery)

Innervation [1] Dorsal branch of the ulnar nerve as a neurocutaneous island flap

Indications [2]
- Defects over the wrist, proximal aspect of the palmar and dorsal hand, and hypothenar area

Contraindications [2]
- Preexisting injuries to the wrist and distal forearm area

Advantages [2]
- Constant anatomy
- Simple and reliable
- Large vessel diameter
- Long pedicle
- Good and large arc of rotation
- Sensate

Disadvantages [2]
- Possible loss of ulnar artery with future cold intolerance (standard flap technique)
- Paresthesia in the area supplied by ulnar nerve

N. Alohaideb (✉)
Plastic Surgery Division, Department of Surgery, Ministry of National Guard - Health Affairs, King Abdullah International Medical Research Center, Riyadh, Saudi Arabia

O. Almeshal et al. (eds.), *Soft Tissue Reconstruction of the Hand: Loco-regional and Distant Flaps Selection and Approach*,
https://doi.org/10.1007/978-981-16-9945-0_37

- Visually exposed donor site
- Hair growth in recipient site
- Increased fracture risk in case of bone harvest
- Postoperative lymphatic edema

Marking Technique [2–7]

- The patient is placed in a supine position with the arm abducted on the arm table.
- The technique can be performed under general anesthesia or regional anesthesia with the use of a tourniquet without exsanguination.
- Before the beginning of marking, Allen's test is required to confirm the continuity of the palmar arch.
- Pisiform eminence is marked; then, a line is drawn from this point to the medial epicondyle of the humerus, which represents the midline of the flap.
- The flap is centered around a point 4–7 cm proximal to the pisiform eminence along the axis drawn over the ulna.
- The dorsal branch of the ulnar artery is located between the flexor carpi ulnaris muscle and the extensor carpi ulnaris muscle about 2–4 cm from the pisiform eminence (Fig. 37.1).
- The dorsal branch of the ulnar artery should be identified and marked using Doppler ultrasound.
- The flap is marked according to the defect size with a width not exceeding that of the palmaris longus muscle tendon palmarly and extensor digitorum communis muscle tendon dorsally; the length should not exceed two-thirds of the length of the ulnar forearm.
- The rotation point of the flap is about 2–4 cm from a pisiform eminence, depending on the origin of the dorsal branch from the ulnar artery.

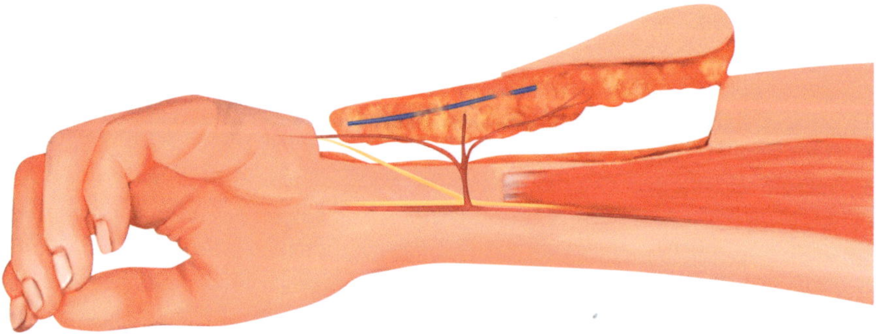

Fig. 37.1 The location of the dorsal branch of the ulnar artery, which is located about 2–4 cm from the pisiform eminence and is usually found between the flexor carpi ulnaris muscle and the extensor carpi ulnaris muscle. The dorsal branch of the ulnar nerve is in the vicinity of the pedicle and should be protected

Surgical Technique [2, 3, 8, 9]

- After marking is complete, the incision is made through the skin and then the fascia around the marked flap.
- Few skin sutures to fasciae are applied to stabilize the flap.
- Dissection is made starting from the radial side in the plane between fascia and paratenon of the tendon or the perimysium of the muscle of flexor carpi ulnaris.
- Once reaching the lateral border of flexor carpi ulnaris, suitable perforators will be visualized arising from the septum between the flexor carpi ulnaris and the flexor digitorum superficialis.
- Perforators are traced until the origin from the ulnar artery; the inclusion of a cuff of muscle around these perforators is advised in order not to damage them.
- The dorsal ulnar nerve should be identified and dissected away from the pedicle to preserve it.
- At this moment, the ulnar artery is clamped and the tourniquet is deflated to check for hand perfusion.
- The tourniquet is again inflated and complete dissection proximally to distally until reaching the pivot point 2 cm from the pisiform bone is done.
- Preserving a skin bridge distally will reduce the chance of lowered perfusion or venous stasis.
- Then, tourniquet is released and flap perfusion is checked.
- Hemostasis is achieved; then, the flap is turned accordingly with a rotation of 100 degrees and 270 degrees.
- The donor area is closed primarily if possible or with STSG.

Postop Care [2]

- Wrist immobilization in 30-degree extension with volar forearm splint for 10–14 days
- Initiation of physical therapy and scar management after complete flap healing

Complications [7]

- Flap tip necrosis
- Complete flap necrosis
- Venous congestion
- Infection

Variants

- Dorsal ulnar artery perforator fascia flap
- Dorsal ulnar artery perforator free flap
- Dorsal ulnar neurocutaneous island flap [1]
- Dorsal ulnar artery osteofasciocutaneous flap [10]

Case

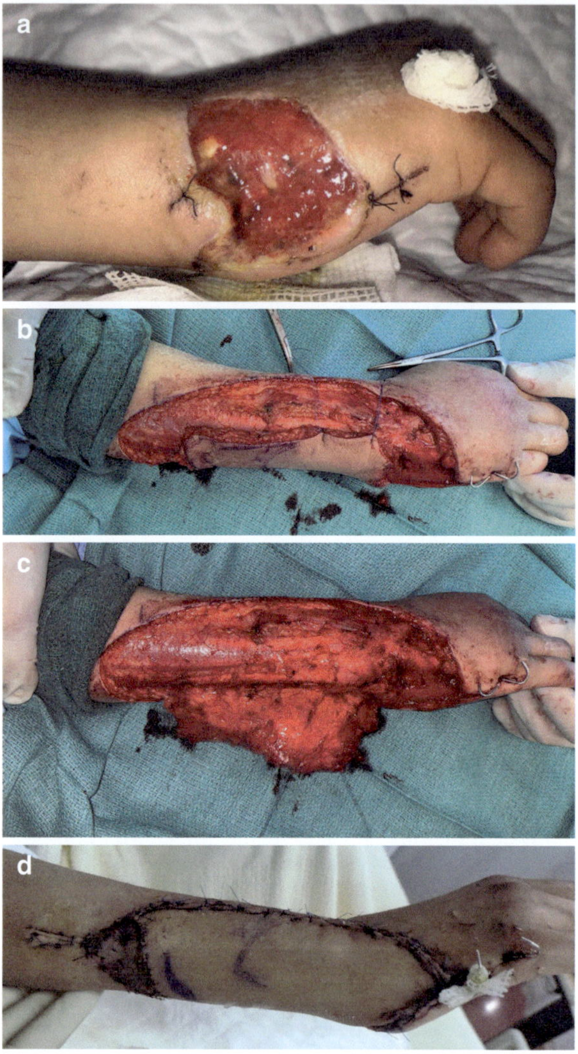

Case 37.1 Preoperative photo of a patient who presented with ulnar-sided hand and wrist wound with exposed underlying bone after she received initial trauma management in another institute, shown in (**a**). Coverage with dorsal ulnar artery perforator flap was planned after identifying the perforators with handheld Doppler. The flap was elevated as seen in (**b**) with preservation of ulnar artery perforator as seen in (**c**). The flap was then advanced to cover the hand and wrist defect and the raw donor area was skin-grafted as seen in (**d**)

References

1. Ülkür E, Açikel C, Eren F, Çeliköz B. Use of dorsal ulnar neurocutaneous island flap in the treatment of chronic postburn palmar contractures. Burns. 2005;31(1):99–104.
2. Hierner R, Putz R, Bishop AT, Shen Z, Wilhelm K. Flaps in hand and upper limb reconstruction: surgical anatomy, operative techniques, and differential therapy. 2014.
3. Krishnan KG. An illustrated handbook of flap-raising techniques. Stuttgart: Thieme; 2008.
4. Martinez FM, Navarro MLG, Navarro JG, Ros AG, Robledano AI. Hand coverage. In: Amr S, editor. Issues in flap surgery. InTech; 2018.
5. Chao JD, Huang JM, Wiedrich TA. Local hand flaps. J Am Soc Surg Hand. 2001;1(1):25–44.
6. Antonopoulos D, Kang NV, Debono R. Our experience with the use of the dorsal ulnar artery flap in hand and wrist tissue cover. J Hand Surg. 1997;22(6):739–44.
7. Khan MM, Yaseen M, Bariar L, Khan SM. Clinical study of dorsal ulnar artery flap in hand reconstruction. Indian J Plastic Surg. 2009;42(1):52.
8. Karacalar A, Özcan M. Preliminary report: the distally pedicled dorsoulnar forearm flap for hand reconstruction. Br J Plastic Surg. 1999;52(6):453–7.
9. Karacalar A, Özcan M. Department of technique use of a subcutaneous pedicle ulnar flap to cover skin defects around the wrist. J Hand Surg. 1998;23(3):551–5. https://doi.org/10.1016/S0363-5023(05)80478-2.
10. Choupina M, Malheiro E, Guimarães I, Pinho C, Silva P, Ferreira P, Reis J, Amarante J. Osteofasciocutaneous flap based on the dorsal ulnar artery. a new option for reconstruction of composite hand defects. Br J Plastic Surg. 2004;57(5):465–8.

Part VI

Pedicled Flaps: Distant Flaps

Thoracoabdominal Flap

38

Ali I. Hadadi and Nawaf Alohaideb

Classification [1, 2] Fasciocutaneous flap, type C

Vascular Supply [1, 2]
- *Dominant pedicle*: rectus abdominis muscle myocutaneous perforators (*superior epigastric artery*)
- *Minor pedicle*: 2–3 subcostal arteries

Innervation [1, 2] Anterior division of 6th–10th intercostal nerves

Indications [2–5]
- Ipsilateral upper extremity defects
- Abdomen, anterior thorax, and breast defects
- Cloacal exstrophy

Contraindications [1–3]
- Perforator to thoracoepigastric flap usually jeopardized if inframammary fold is violated preoperatively, making this flap unreliable

Advantages [1, 2]
- Technical ease
- Donor site closed primarily
- Hidden scar

A. I. Hadadi · N. Alohaideb (✉)
Plastic Surgery Division, Department of Surgery, Ministry of National Guard – Health Affairs, King Abdullah International Medical Research Center, Riyadh, Saudi Arabia

O. Almeshal et al. (eds.), *Soft Tissue Reconstruction of the Hand: Loco-regional and Distant Flaps Selection and Approach*,
https://doi.org/10.1007/978-981-16-9945-0_38

Disadvantages [1, 2]

- Random blood supply to the distal portion, making blood supply unreliable.

Marking Technique [1, 2]

- The patient is placed in a supine position (Fig. 38.1).
- The flap width is extended between the xiphoid and another point 7 cm below the xiphoid.

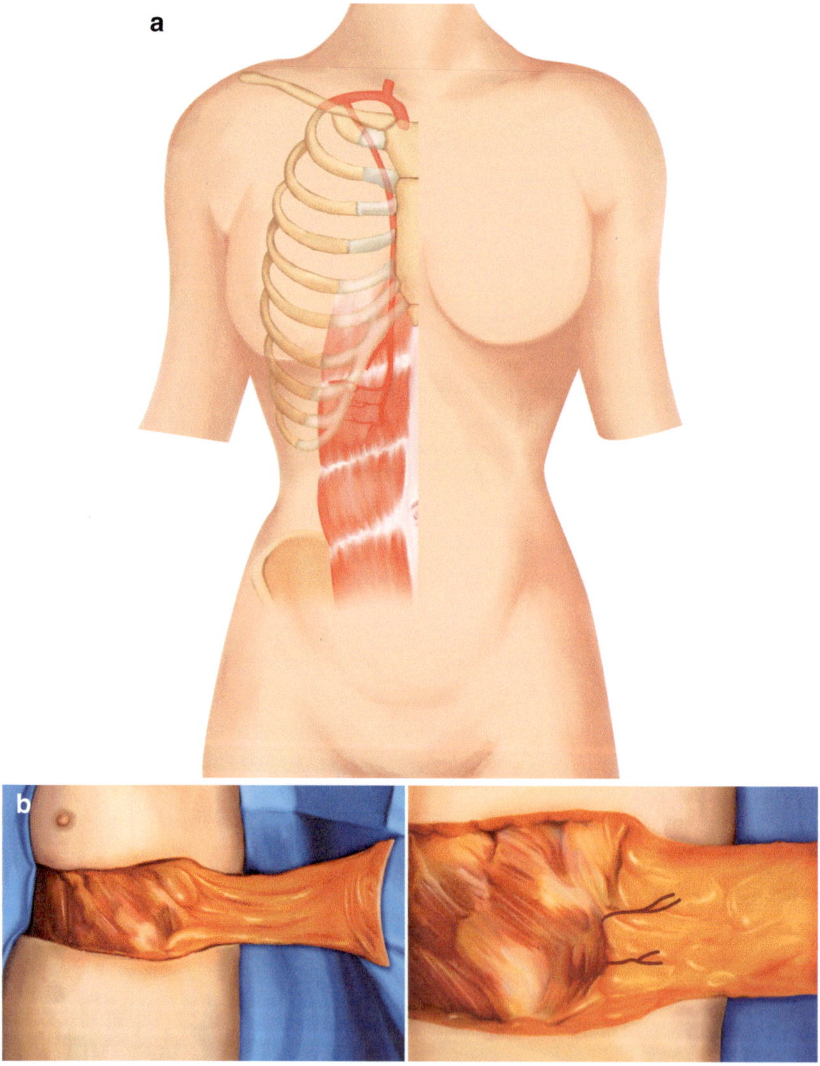

Fig. 38.1 (**a**) The locations of the superior epigastric artery and its perforators in which the flap is based on. The flap was designed after palpating and locating the xiphoid to represent the upper limit of the flap. The other line is about 7 cm below the first line and is based on skin pinch to assess donor elasticity and the ability to close the donor site primely. The perforators are located with the aid of handheld Doppler. The flap is then elevated on the suprafascial plane till the perforators are located and protected as seen in (**b**)

- Marking is done by drawing two lines: the first line started at the xiphoid and the other parallel line 7 cm below it across the lateral flank with the two lines joined as rectangular or elliptical termination over the lateral flank.

Surgical Technique [1, 2]

- Incision is made utilizing the two lines with lateral to medial dissection.
- The flap tip is raised immediately superficial to the serratus and external oblique fascial layers laterally with dissection continuing until the linea semilunaris is reached medially.
- Dissection beyond linea semilunaris medially is critical because it might damage the perforator, rendering the flap ischemic.
- The flap tip beyond the anterior axillary line is not reliable, and vascular delay (3–7 days) is recommended before flap elevation to enhance the blood supply.
- Back cut through the skin only (i.e., not full thickness to preserve the inferior perforators) can be utilized to enhance the arc of rotation.
- The flap is always transferred as a pedicle; therefore, excessive tension or kinking should be avoided to preserve the fragile perforators.
- The flap is inset into the recipient site with absorbable sutures in two layers with the fascia of Scarpa being the deep layer.
- Closed suction drains are inserted.
- The donor site is closed primarily with the repair of the fascia of Scarpa; however, if this is not feasible, a skin graft can be used for coverage.

Postop Care [1, 2]

- Ambulation is allowed 1–2 days postop and standing straight around 3–4 days postop.

Complications [1, 2]

- Wound healing impairment (due to random blood supply)
- Infection

Variants N/A

References

1. Reconstructive surgery, anatomy, techniques and clinical applications Ch.10E. p. 1270–78.
2. Brown RG, Vasconez LO, Jurkiewicz MJ. Transverse abdominal flaps and the deep epigastric arcade. Plast Reconstr Surg. 1975;55:416–21.
3. Davis WD, McCraw JB, Carraway JH. Use of a direct transverse, thoracoabdominal flap to close difficult wounds of the thorax and upper extremity. Plast Reconstr Surg. 1977;60:526–33.
4. Lewis VL Jr, Cook JQ. The nondelayed thoracoepigastric flap: coverage of an extensive electric burn defect of the upper extremity. Plast Reconstr Surg. 1980;65:492–3.
5. Schaeffer CS, King LR, Levin LS. Use of the expanded thoracoepigastric myocutaneous flap in the closure of cloacal exstrophy. Plast Reconstr Surg. 1996 Jun;97(7):1479–84.

Abdominal Flap

39

Ali I. Hadadi and Nawaf Alohaideb

Classification [1] Fasciocutaneous flap

Vascular Supply [1] Subdermal plexus supplied by periumbilical perforator arising from the interconnection between the deep inferior epigastric artery and the intercostal arteries

Innervation [1, 2] Subdermal plexus of thoracoabdominal, lateral cutaneous, subcostal, iliohypogastric, and ilioinguinal nerves

Indications [3, 4]
- Pediatric (aged less than 2 years) complex hand defects
- Preparation of toe-to-hand transfers by coverage of digital stump defects
- High-voltage electric burns of the hands
- Mutilating hand injuries
- Length preservation in case of multiple digital amputations
- Lack of microsurgical expertise

Contraindication [1, 5–7]
- Donor area within the zone of injury
- Preexisting scar in adjacent tissue
- Obese abdominal wall (compromises the vascular supply)
- Inability for immobilization for 3 weeks
- Large defect
- Defect with a greater arc of rotation required

A. I. Hadadi · N. Alohaideb (✉)
Plastic Surgery Division, Department of Surgery, Ministry of National Guard - Health Affairs, King Abdullah International Medical Research Center, Riyadh, Saudi Arabia

O. Almeshal et al. (eds.), *Soft Tissue Reconstruction of the Hand: Loco-regional and Distant Flaps Selection and Approach*,
https://doi.org/10.1007/978-981-16-9945-0_39

Advantages [1, 3, 4]

- Technical ease
- Lack of microvascular anastomosis
- Donor site closed primarily
- Hidden scar

Disadvantages [1, 3, 4]

- Random blood supply to the distal portion
- Two-stage procedure with the need of flap separation
- Patient discomfort
- Joint stiffness
- Increased hospital length of stay
- Need for flap debulking

Marking Technique [1, 3, 4]

- The patient is placed in a supine position.
- The axis of the flap is based on paraumbilical perforators identified by the Doppler signal (Fig. 39.1).
- The average length to width ratio of 3:1 (approximately 6–8 cm in width and 28–30 cm in length) can be utilized.
- The lateral limit of the flap is a posterior axillary line and the medial limit is linea semilunaris.

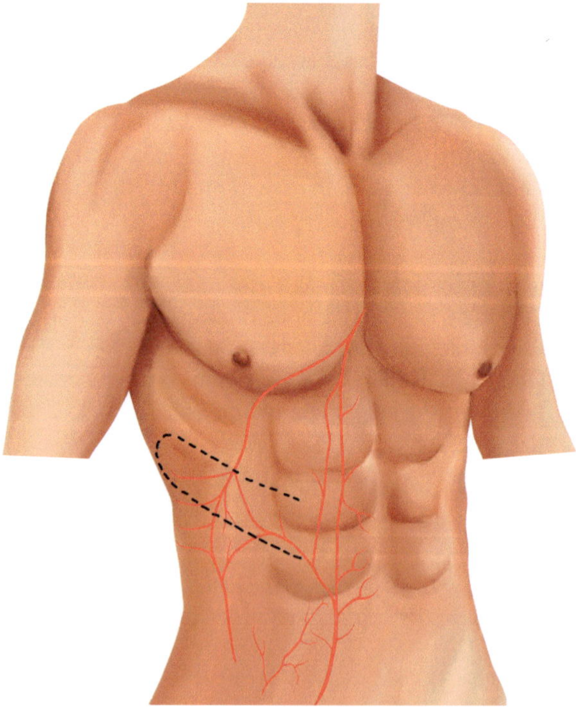

Fig. 39.1 The flap design that is based on paraumbilical perforators. The perforators are located with the aid of a handheld Doppler and the flap is designed based on that

Surgical Technique [1, 3, 4]

- The incision is made utilizing the marking with lateral to medial dissection.
- The flap tip is raised in the suprafascial plane of the external oblique muscle laterally with dissection continuing to base the pedicle of the flap on the lateral border of the rectus abdominis muscle, that is, until the linea semilunaris is encountered medially.
- The dissection in the loose areolar plane can be performed by electrocautery or sharp dissection.
- Subfascial dissection should be avoided before linea semilunaris is reached medially.
- The fascia of Scarpa at the flap margins should be dissected, and a small perforator is either ligated or dissected with electrocautery while raising the flap.
- The lateral margin of the flap is dissected elliptically to facilitate the primary closure.
- Once the linea semilunaris is encountered medially, the dissection is stopped in the suprafascial plane.
- If the defect size is large, an incision of linea semilunaris and inclusion of the rectus abdominis muscle can be performed.
- The closure was performed in two layers (deep layer and skin) with absorbable monofilament or braided 3–0 interrupted suture used for deep-layered closure, and skin closure is kept according to the surgeon's preference.
- The flap is inset into the recipient site with monofilament 3–0 or 4–0 permanent interrupted technique.
- The distal end of the flap is inset without tension.
- The pedicle end of the flap (proximal end) is kept as an open acute wound.
- Dressing for all wounds was performed by nonadherent gauze followed by bulky dry gauze.
- After the dressing, immobilization and support of the upper extremity to the trunk are performed.
- The flap separation and pedicle division are commonly performed in 3 weeks and can be delayed to 4–5 weeks if vascular ingrowth is not optimal or the patient has comorbidity delaying the wound healing.
- The pedicle is divided sharply, and the donor area is closed primarily after securing the hemostasis.

Postop Care [1, 3]

- Ambulation at 1–2 days postop and standing straight around 3–4 days postop
- Dressing changes as per the surgeon's preference

Complications [1, 3, 4]

- Infection
- Partial of full flap necrosis
- Wound dehiscence.

Variants [1, 8]

- Paraumbilical perforator flap
- Thoracoumbilical flap

Case

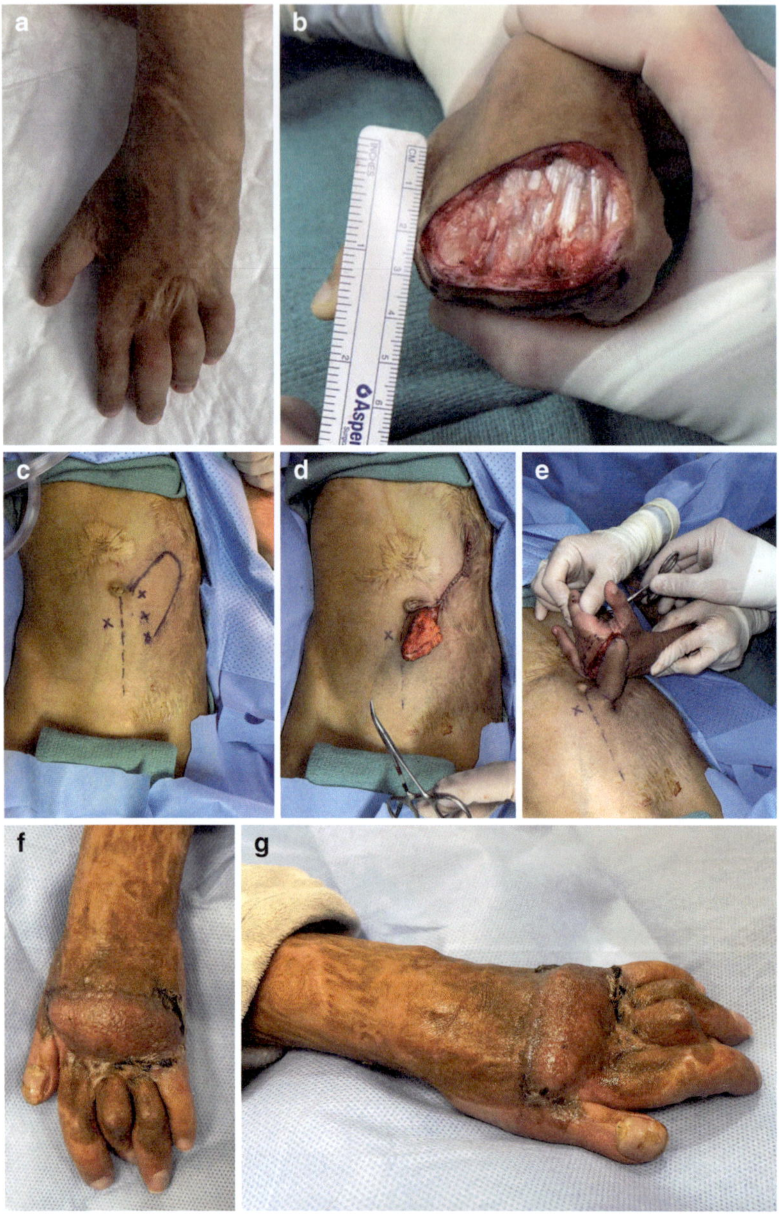

Case 39.1 A 9-year-old patient presented with a left-hand burn contracture in extension position as seen in (**a**). The preoperative assessment of general body scars that involved most of the upper limb and trunk was performed. Release of contracture yielded a hand dorsum defect with exposed extensor tendons as shown in (**b**). Paraumbilical perforator flap was planned in which the perforators were mapped with handheld Doppler with flap being designed to the dimensions of the hand defect as in (**c**). Flap was then raised making sure to preserve the perforators as in (**d**); then, it was inset over the hand defect as in (**e**) after ensuring proper alignment of the hand defect and the flap. The flap was left attached for 3 weeks, after which it was divided as shown in (**f**). Follow-up of the patient 1 month after the flap division is seen in (**g**)

References

1. Gutwein LG, Merrell GA, Knox KR. Paraumbilical perforator flap for soft tissue reconstruction of the forearm. J Hand Surg Am. 2015;40(3):586–92.
2. Jelinek LA, Gogna S, Ferguson T. Anatomy, abdomen and pelvis, anterolateral abdominal wall fascia. 2017.
3. Al-Qattan MM, Al-Qattan AM. Defining the indications of pedicled groin and abdominal flaps in hand reconstruction in the current microsurgery era. J Hand Surg Am. 2016;41(9):917–27.
4. Goertz O, Kapalschinski N, Daigeler A, Hirsch T, Homann HH, Steinstraesser L, Lehnhardt M, Steinau HU. The effectiveness of pedicled groin flaps in the treatment of hand defects: results of 49 patients. J Hand Surg Am. 2012;37(10):2088–94.
5. Choudry UH, Moran SL, Li S, et al. Soft tissue coverage of the elbow: an outcome analysis and reconstructive algorithm. Plast Reconstr Surg. 2007;119:1852–7.
6. Herter F, Ninkovic M, Ninkovic M. Rational flap selection and timing for coverage of complex upper extremity trauma. J Plast Reconstr Aesthet Surg. 2007;60:760–8.
7. Hallock GG. The utility of both muscle and fascia flaps in severe upper extremity trauma. J Trauma. 2002;53:61–5.
8. Naalla R, De M, Dawar R, Chauhan S, Singhal M. Thoracoumbilical flap: anatomy, technique, and clinical applications in upper limb reconstruction in the era of microvascular surgery. J Hand Microsurg. 2018;10(1):29–36.

Groin Flap

40

Ali I. Hadadi and Nawaf Alohaideb

Classification [1] Fasciocutaneous flap, type A

Vascular Supply [1] Superficial circumflex iliac artery

Innervation [1] T12 lateral cutaneous nerve

Indications [2] Hand and forearm wound coverage as pedicled flap

Contraindications [2] Groin cancer or previous radiotherapy, anatomical malformation, or previous groin surgery

Advantages [3]
- Technical ease
- Constant vascular anatomy (superficial circumflex iliac artery)
- Upper limb defect coverage without microvascular anastomosis

Disadvantages [3]
- Two-stage procedure in upper limb reconstruction
- Discomfort and stiffness of the elbow and hand in pedicle groin
- Thick flap requiring defatting with a less aesthetic appearance

---

A. I. Hadadi · N. Alohaideb (✉)
Plastic Surgery Division, Department of Surgery, Ministry of National Guard - Health Affairs, King Abdullah International Medical Research Center, Riyadh, Saudi Arabia

O. Almeshal et al. (eds.), *Soft Tissue Reconstruction of the Hand: Loco-regional and Distant Flaps Selection and Approach*,
https://doi.org/10.1007/978-981-16-9945-0_40

Marking Technique [1]

- The patient is placed in a supine position with the posterior iliac spine on the ipsilateral side of the flap harvest elevated by a beanbag to assist in flap harvest (Fig. 40.1).

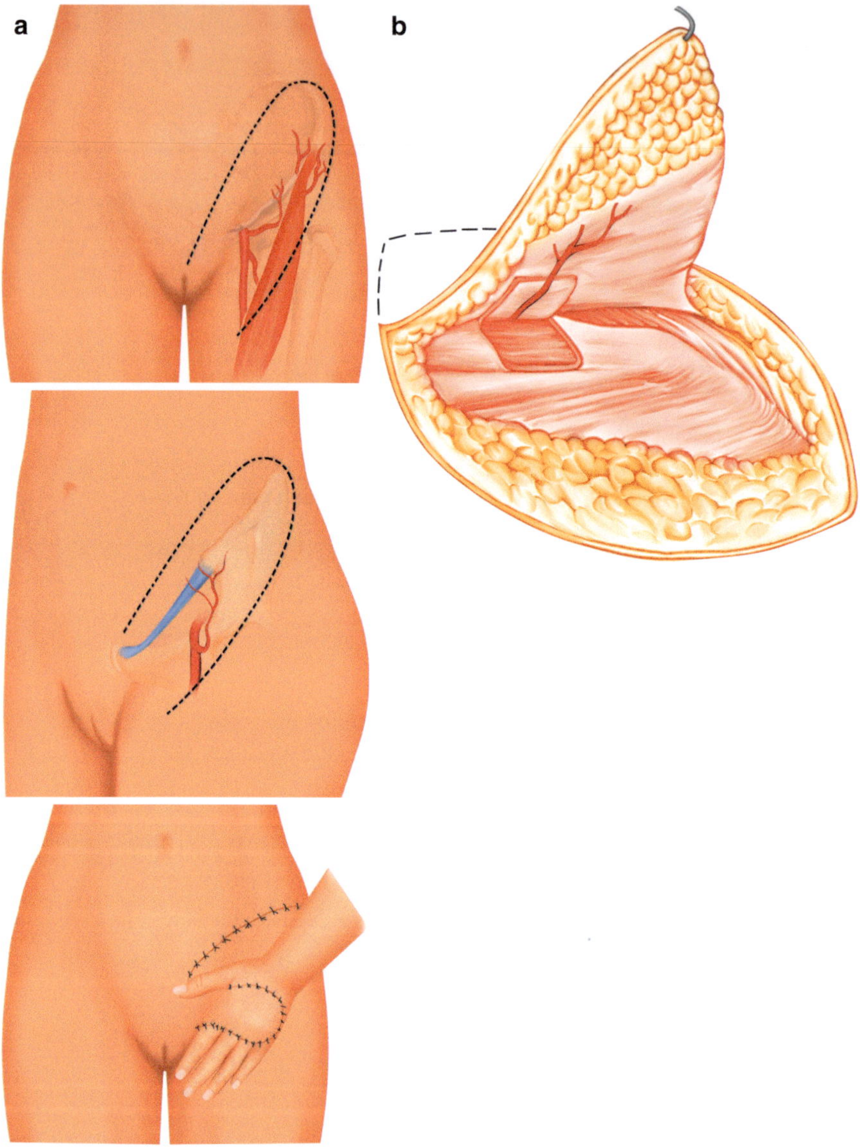

Fig. 40.1 (**a**) The marking of the flap in which the anterior superior iliac spine and pubic tubercle are marked with an imaginary line in between that corresponds to the inguinal ligament. The flap periphery there is marked to include the area 1/3 above and 2/3 below the inguinal ligament. The sartorius muscle is then marked in which its medial aspect is also marked. The flap inset is shown in which the ipsilateral hand is bent and the flap is inset into the hand soft tissue defect. (**b**) The transition point of flap elevation and dissection point in which at the medial edge of the sartorius muscle, subfascial plane of elevation is done to include the flap pedicle

- Marking is done by drawing a line between the pubic tubercle and the anterior superior iliac spine overlying the inguinal ligament.
- Flap width is measured by the rule of thirds, 1/3 (or two fingerbreadths) above the line and 2/3 below, which is around 3 cm superior and 6 cm inferior to the inguinal ligament.
- The pedicle is found 3 cm below and parallel to the inguinal ligament, marked under Doppler guidance.

Surgical Technique [1]

- After marking is complete, incision is made through the superior, inferior, and lateral margins superficial to fascia lata distally to proximally, that is, from the ASIS distally until the medial border of sartorius muscle is reached proximally. Then, the dissection continues deep to investing fascia and superficial to sartorius muscle to avoid injury to the pedicle.
- Vascular pedicle in the femoral triangle is identified.
- The flap can be utilized as transposition, tubed pedicled, or free flap.
- The point of rotation from the femoral vessel below the inguinal ligament is used to cover the abdominal defect, perineum, or upper extremity.
- For the delay of groin flap, the abovementioned steps are followed with a few modifications:
  - The upper and lower incisions are lengthened (i.e., equal to the width of the flap).
  - The distal incision is not performed.
  - The flap is undermined to the medial border of the sartorius.
  - Flap distal incision can be performed after 10–14 days.
- Flap transfer depends on the flap variant used:
  - A standard flap transferred directly to the defect with a back cut is used to increase the arc of rotation.
  - Tubed pedicle flap is transferred as delay flap requiring separation after 2–3 weeks.
  - Island flap is transferred under the tunnel.
- The flap is inset with removing the excess subcutaneous tissue lateral to the sartorius and sutured to the edge of the defect directly or tubed proximal portion as in upper extremity defect.
- The donor site is closed primarily whenever possible or with a skin graft if needed.

Postop Care [1]

- The wrist is sutured to torso to help prevent flap dehiscence once the patient is fully awake.
- Ambulation is allowed 1–2 days postop and standing straight around 3–4 days.

Complications [3]

- Partial necrosis
- Infection
- Seroma

Variants [1]

- Delay flap
- Island flap
- Free flap.

Case

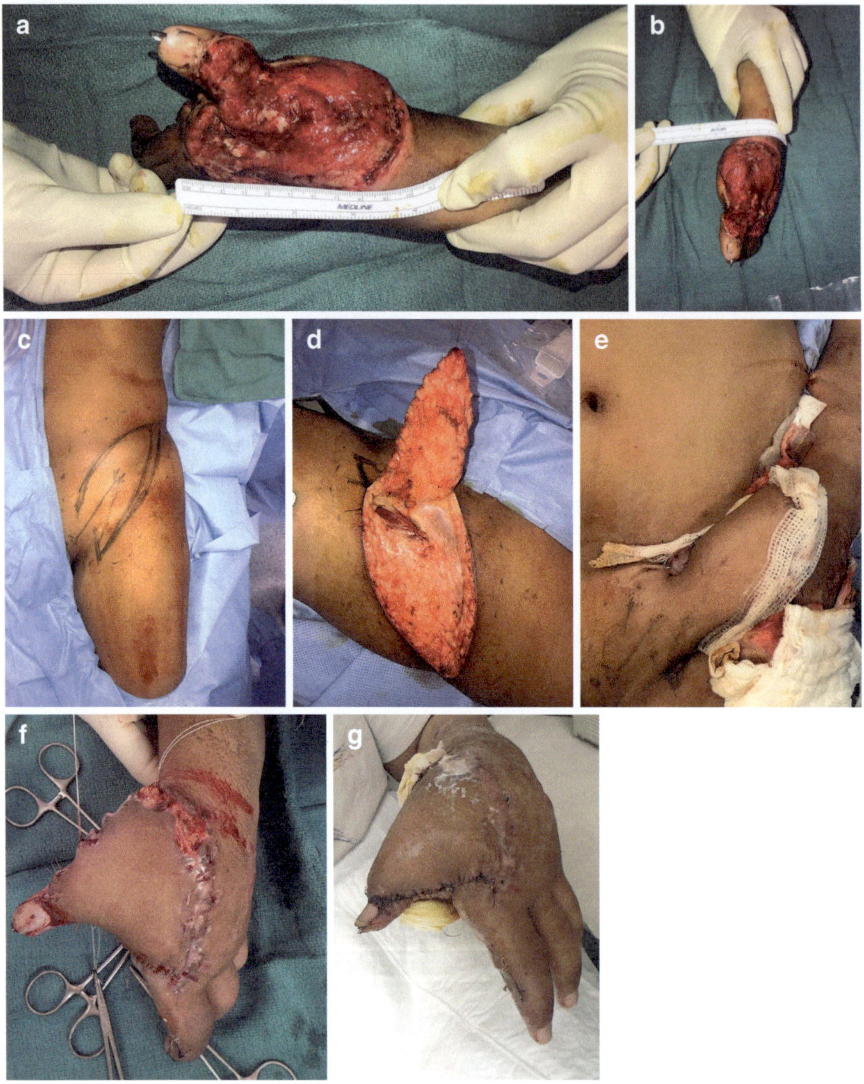

Case 40.1 Intraoperative photos of a patient with thumb soft tissue defect with the exposed bone are seen in (**a**) and (**b**). After wound irrigation and debridement, the wound was ready for soft tissue coverage in which a groin flap was planned. (**c**) The marking of the flap on the patient's left groin. The flap was raised distally to proximally in the suprafascial plane till identifying the lateral edge of the sartorius muscle, after which subfascial dissection was carried out as seen in (**d**). The flap was then inset to the defect after ensuring proper coverage of the defect as in (**e**). The flap was left attached for a period of 3 weeks; then, it was divided as in (**f**). Follow-up of the patient one month after the flap division is seen in (**g**)

References

1. Reconstructive surgery, anatomy, techniques and clinical applications, Ch.10E. p. 1245–62.
2. Amouzou KS, Berny N, El Harti A, Diouri M, Chlihi A, Ezzoubi M. The pedicled groin flap in resurfacing hand burn scar release and other injuries: a five-case series report and review of the literature. Ann Burns Fire Disasters. 2017;30(1):57–61.
3. Arner M, Möller K. Morbidity of the pedicled groin flap. A retrospective study of 44 cases. Scand J Plast Reconstr Surg Hand Surg. 1994;28(2):143–6.

Index

O. Almeshal et al. (eds.), *Soft Tissue Reconstruction of the Hand: Loco-regional and Distant Flaps Selection and Approach*,
https://doi.org/10.1007/978-981-16-9945-0

MIX
Papier aus verantwortungsvollen Quellen
Paper from responsible sources
FSC® C105338

If you have any concerns about our products,
you can contact us on
ProductSafety@springernature.com

In case Publisher is established outside the EU,
the EU authorized representative is:
Springer Nature Customer Service Center GmbH
Europaplatz 3, 69115 Heidelberg, Germany

Printed by Libri Plureos GmbH
in Hamburg, Germany